Developing and Using Quality Indicators
For Emergency Medical Services
Evaluation and Improvement

I0470873

Craig A. Stroup

Center for EMS Performance Improvement
ISBN#978-1491251522
www.cemspi.org

Developing and Using Quality Indicators
For Emergency Medical Services
Evaluation and Improvement

Contents

Developing and Using Quality Indicators
For Emergency Medical Services
Evaluation and Improvement

Contents - Continued

FOREWORD

With the ever changing healthcare environment surrounding the Emergency Medical Services (EMS) Industry today, now more than ever EMS professionals need to be able to show what their systems are doing and how well they are doing it. This is the true utility and purpose of a quality indicator.

Whether you call them benchmarks, measures, metrics, markers or indicators, understanding how to capture and present EMS system performance information is often a difficult but important task.

While there are many paths which lead to a high performance quality improvement program, an integral part of any program is the collection and conversion of raw data to information and then to meaningful and simple communication between the users of the system. Integrating quality indicators should be a common theme in any and all quality programs.

This book focuses on helping Continuous Quality Improvement professionals with a very important part of their comprehensive EMS-CQI program; the closing of the gap between collecting data and acting on it. The book can be used as a textbook companion to an organized training program and includes demonstrations, exercises, templates and other tools to facilitate the utilization of EMS performance oriented quality indicators.

PART I

Putting Things in Perspective

Putting Things in Perspective

When all is said and done, the concepts of quality improvement are mostly about motivating groups of people with common interests to do their best. Not really a new concept. In fact, sports teams have been doing this for many years. It's an accepted conclusion that some will do very well and others not so well. But what is not so accepted is when a very talented team underachieves, or when a team with a clear lack of talent overachieves. These are the opportunities where the concepts of continuous quality improvement (CQI) come into the picture. In much the same way that coaches and players have for years collected and evaluated information by films and statistics, CQI collects information in the form of data and in the same tradition tries to motivate the team to perform better by looking at themselves and setting goals for improvement. (27)

Quality Indicators are the films and statistics of CQI programs. The data by itself has very little if any value. It is the veritable sleeping tiger. Unless we wake it we are indifferent to it and it has little if any concern for us. Data has to be transformed into a meaningful format. This is what we call an "Indicator". Quality Indicators, which are sometimes called measures, metrics, benchmarks, as well as other terms depending upon the nature of their use, are the "growl of the Sabertooth." They are the signal which stimulates us and tell us whether we should get up and run or simply go back to sleep.

If American industry defines quality as "the degree of which a system is free from bugs and flaws" (5), then it would seem that Emergency Medical Services (EMS) as a relatively young industry appears to be at a tolerable level. But if we were to be completely truthful with ourselves considering all that we have learned about today's EMS systems and the expectations of our customers, the answer is probably closer to; "we don't really know". Even though we have been around for fifty plus years, comparably we are a very young industry and profession. This is our role. To recognize, communicate and improve on activities like: field assessments, dosage errors, scene times and cardiac arrest save rates. These are just some of our common challenges.

Although the main concepts of CQI focus on the process, in the end it is more about the people who perform those processes. While it is true that the activities surrounding CQI primarily focus on measuring processes and outcomes, the real action is when these measures communicate well to a group and ultimately stimulate the discussion and motivation to get a group of people to believe that they can make something better. The process is full circle when a group of stakeholders and experts all agree to work together to produce an outcome that has value to all.

Traditional Continuous Quality Improvement (CQI) Model

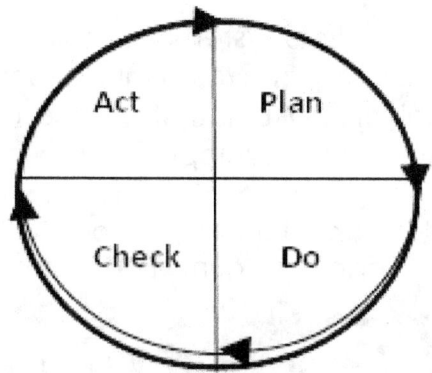

Historically, the traditional model for quality improvement has focused on a four phased Plan-Do-Check-Act (PDCA) model which leads organizations through a cycle of improvement. Quality Indicators tend to be primarily a part of the "check" phase where stakeholders are interested in evaluating system performance.

The EMS Quality Manger

Today's EMS quality programs need highly capable people who can do incredible things. Unfortunately, many EMS provider and governmental agencies struggle to find their quality program identity and are often confused about how a true quality program operates within an efficient EMS system. This often leads to quality improvement programs that are underfunded and exist within an organization in name only remaining a low priority. [26] [28]

Moreover, it is not uncommon for EMS organizations to designate their highest performing data person, paramedic, nurse or a physician as the head of their quality program with little or no experience or training for this critical role. [24] This situation often results in the default old school quality assurance model where random charts are reviewed for compliance and interaction with providers is limited to what didn't go well for the individual care provider. This is not to say that the individual patient safety event should not be reviewed; on the contrary important system catch points and monitoring of EMS patient safety events should be a constant within all EMS Systems. But individual provider performance reviews such as those related to a patient safety event should be limited to a separate process or as part of a separate patient safety program. It is important to also recognize that trends that are identified through a patient safety program may be the starting point for a broader and system-wide quality review or initiative.

Mixing the responsibilities of quality consensus building with individual performance review and safety events - sets the Quality Manger up with what may be viewed as a negative/punitive experience and may spread to the community making it difficult to motivate and produce positive and effective change. Although patient safety and quality improvement programs are directly related to one another, they have distinctly different processes and approaches to their action models.

7

Integration of Quality Indicators into an EMS System

Whether we realize it or not, most EMS systems are using some sort of quality improvement system within their respective organizations. Some systems are well developed such as the organizational EMS system chart displayed below and others need only some direction to be fully developed.

Actual Organizational Chart for CQI program
California County EMS System

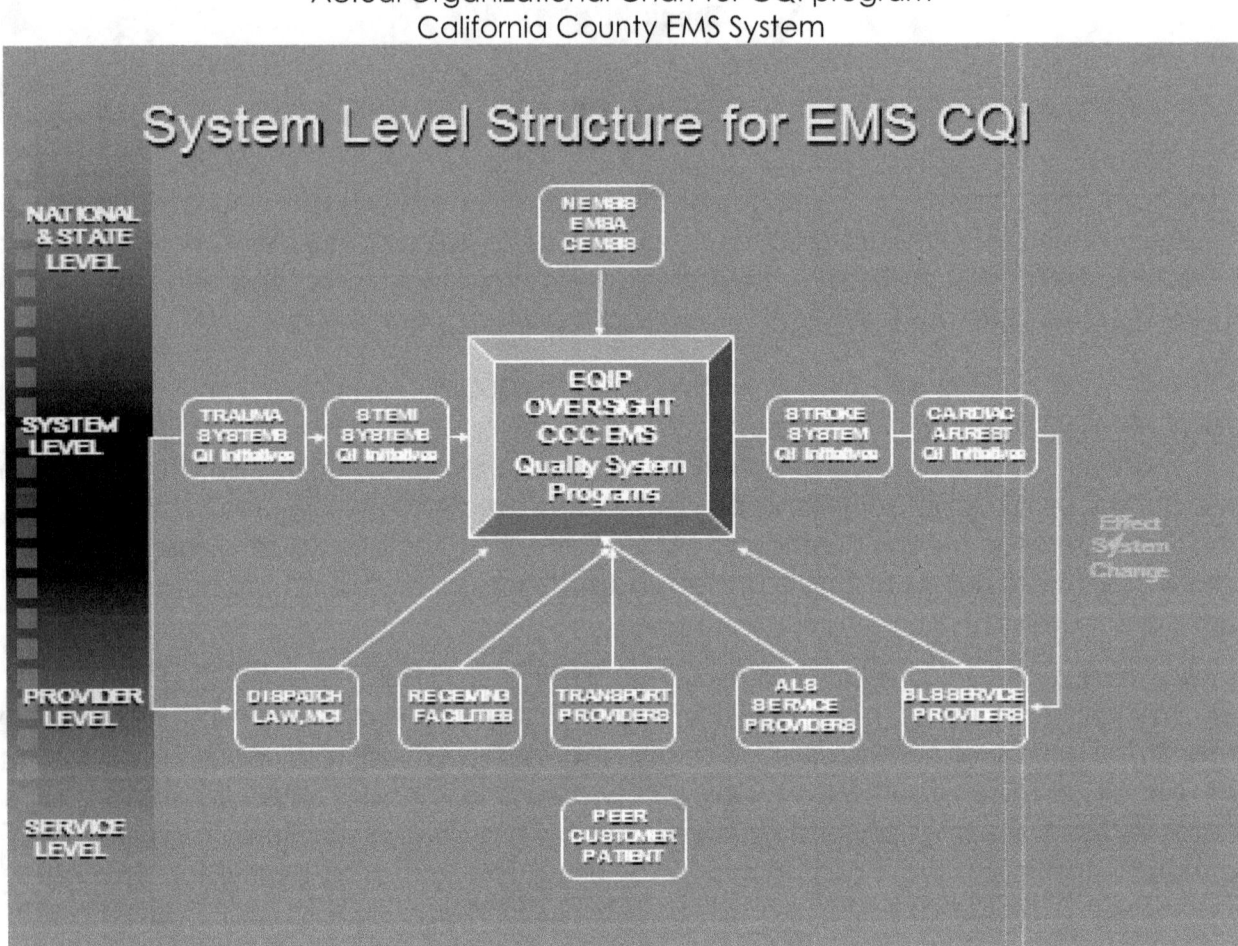

Continual and effective systems have integrated quality indicators as a consensus tool, and have the leadership that reinforces the process and keeps up to date with reporting and continuing education on the overall quality improvement process.

In order to develop and use quality indicators, a consensus network of stakeholders, end users and subject experts must be organized and linked together to drive the quality improvement program. The use of quality indicators within this structure takes hard work and patience on the part of the leadership.

The following link references "Model Guidelines for Quality Improvement in EMS systems" known as document EMSA#166 in California. This document is well developed and may be very applicable to many EMS organizations and Quality Managers. www.emsa.ca.gov/pubs/pdf/emsa166.pdf (11) (27)

The following are examples of actual EMS system indicators regularly reviewed and evaluated by the EMS CQI organization identified in the chart above.

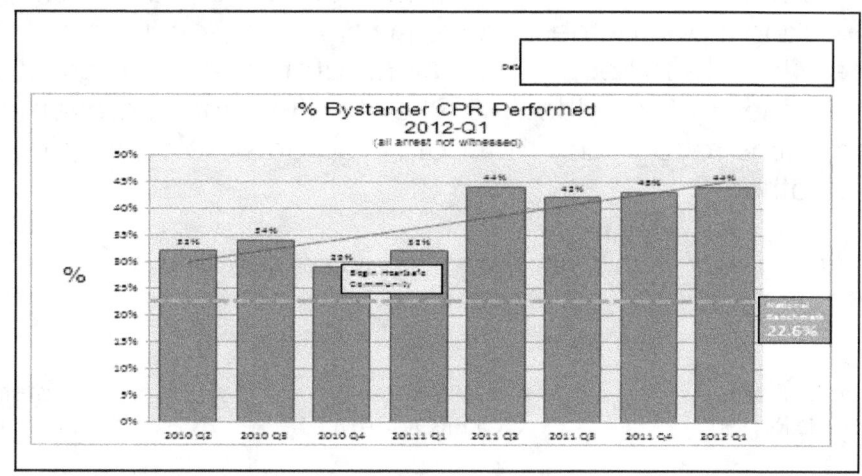

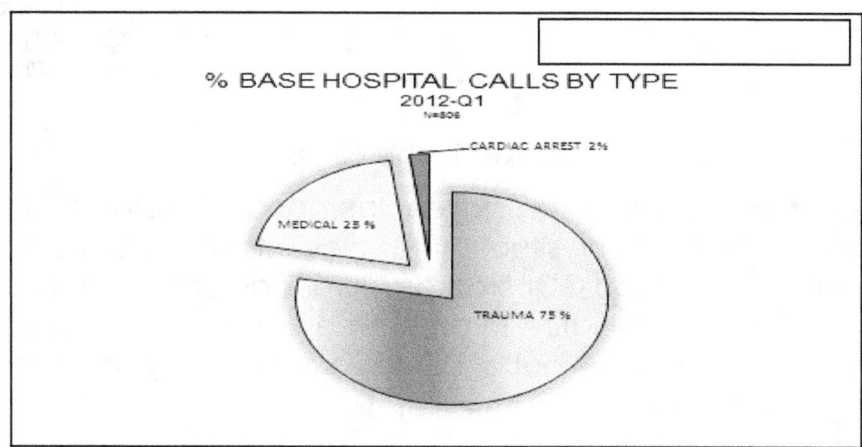

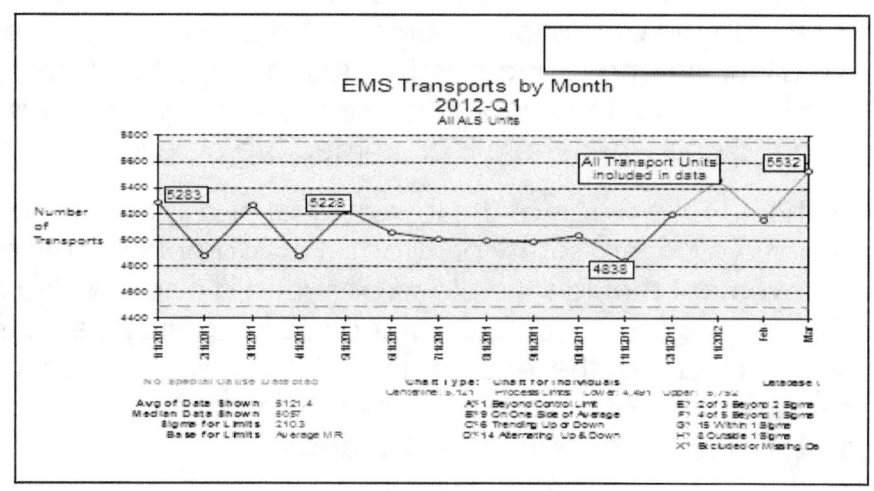

"Old School - New School"

With a new emphasis on patient safety programs, EMS systems and organizations should adopt a model which distinctly separates individual patient safety events from system wide continuous improvement. The vast majority of improvements in patient care come <u>not</u> from reacting to what went wrong, but from discovering what went right and then making it part of the culture. (15) For this reason, Quality Managers should go to great lengths to keep their patient safety events program separate operationally from their system wide EMS-QI evaluation and improvement program. While at the same time recognizing that both programs are equally important and related to one another.

Below is an organizational chart from a functioning EMS system illustrating distinct division between patient safety events reporting programs and the EMS-CQI Program.

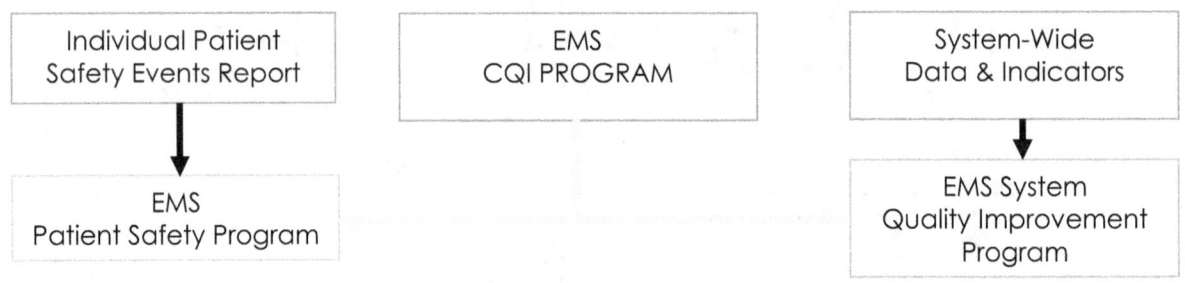

"Snakes in the Grass"

Having a process in place where EMS stakeholders and all customers can be reasonably comfortable reporting situations and events where patient safety is at stake is paramount to any good CQI program. In all cases, patient safety should be monitored for activity and evaluated to determine is indicators should be developed to monitor processes that may be out of control or which may be at unacceptable levels of risk.

Today, traditional "quality assurance' programs where individual cases are routinely reviewed and where corrective "reactions" are taken on a regular basis continue to be more of the rule than the exception. I would argue that this needs to change and trend more towards looking and taking positive action as part of a "systems approach" (27). Individual and singular action is appropriate when it has been discovered or reported and when there is an immediate or serious risk to public safety.

Undoubtedly this should take place at the lowest level of a system food chain and as part of a comprehensive patient safety program. For example; identification of a performance improvement should take place between a captain and firefighter paramedic, ambulance supervisor and paramedic, emergency department RN and paramedic or EMT. If it reaches the level of an EMS agency supervisor or administrator, the issue may have gone too far and is most likely a system issue and may best be handled through system wide CQI analysis.

Below is an example of an actual EMS Policy as part of an EMS agency sponsored Patient Safety Events Reporting Program. The form and a copy of the virtual data screen used to report are located in the resource appendix at the back of this book.

PATIENT SAFETY EVENTS REPORTING PROGRAM POLICY

I. PURPOSE

Patient Safety Events (PSE) are regularly reported and acted upon by the _____ Emergency Medical Services Agency. The purpose of this policy is to provide and identify the process that shall be used to address all PSE. This procedure shall be conducted as a component of the _____ Quality Improvement Process and shall be considered a confidential and protected process of our comprehensive CQI program.

II. POLICY AND PROCEDURE

The following process shall be used to assure that all Patient Safety Events (PSE) are addressed and acted upon by the EMS agency as part of a comprehensive quality improvement and feedback loop for our customers and constituents.

1. Patient Safety Event (PSE) occurs

2. PSE is acknowledged by care givers or other patient advocate

3. PSE Form completed and sent to EMS via email, fax, and mail or by telephone.

4. PSE routed initially to CQI Coordinator for review and assignment.

5. EMS Medical Director and EMS Staff advised of PSE as necessary

5. PSE assigned to appropriate EMS Staff for resolution and follow up.

6. PSE is reviewed by assigned EMS Staff.

7. PSE is evaluated and resolved through CQI process at regularly scheduled Provider Patient-Safety Conferences (**PPC**). (These conferences will be coordinated by EMS and involve a collaborative effort to review, resolve and provide follow up to PSE with only the agencies involved in the event.)

8. PSE resolution or PIP shall be reported to regularly scheduled Internal Patient-Safety Committee (**IPC**)

9. PSE Resolution submitted back to CQI Coordinator for closure

---

Note: Formal training and much more information should be spent on developing a substantial patient safety program within an EMS organization and system. The Center for EMS Performance Improvement (CEMSPI) is a non-profit organization in California which provides training programs, quality oriented resources and tools to assist entities interested in implementing these programs. Their website is; www.cemspi.org.

Developing and Writing a CQI Plan for an EMS Programs

All EMS providers should have a Continuous Quality Improvement plan that describes and sets the foundation for their activity. The EMS CQI Plan should be developed as a simple document that simply describes organization's general CQI plan. A template for this process can be found in the resource appendix at the back of this book. At a minimum, the CQI plan should include a mission statement along with goals and primary objectives of the program. Using a brainstorming technique is an effective way to practice consensus amongst an organization as they develop the plan and fill in the template. The remaining parts of the plan should focus on" what you do?" and "how well do you do it?"

Begin by brainstorming the answers to these questions with your stakeholders and then you're on your way. Take the questions and develop the indicators based upon the answers you are seeking. The organizations core indicators should be identified and be an integral part of the plan. Once the indicators are clearly defined, it is now time to talk to the data people about systems and how you can collect the data to answer these questions.

EMS Data 101

While Quality Managers should be encouraged to be involved in the management of the data system, it is <u>NOT</u> recommended that they take on the dual role of quality and Data System Managers. Instead of punching data entry keys, they should strive to be experts in asking the right questions of their data as well as interpreting and communicating the answers as objectively as possible. With this scope in mind, it becomes incumbent of the Quality Manager to know that his purpose for the data system is to answer quality oriented questions rather than to understand how the data system operates and gathers information. It is best to leave the actual data queries and reporting to the data experts. After all, these are the people who are paid to understand and operate these systems and they are also an important checks and balance in the overall process.

The most important part of what a Quality Manager should know about his data system is how the data will be defined, collected and measured rather than how the machines store and retrieve the data. Quality Mangers should be more about letting "data people" know what it is they want and evaluating the results from a clinical, operational and purely quality point of view. In other words, telling the data system operators "this is what I want – make it happen." The rest should be the data people operating their magic. My observations have been that Quality Managers should be less into data driven systems and much more into "people" driven systems.

So, in fairness to our data people, we need to be clear what we want and how we want it done. So this is where the **quality indicator** becomes such an important tool. It is the tool that marries the data to the chart or table or any reporting format which in the end tells the story about what we have asked. Any good data systems operator will tell you that the results are only as good as the hypothesis. In other words, what goes in - comes out. If you ask for data in a crappy way, you will get a crappy result. It's not the data system operators fault, that is just the basic rule all data systems. They are all perfectly designed for you to get the perfect answer to whatever you ask. So you better ask the right question.

This is the most important value of utilizing a quality indicator. A quality indicator is the tool that you can use to reach consensus on what the clinicians, subject experts or other pertinent stakeholders want to ask as well as what the data operators need to know to obtain and produce the answers. The indicators provide what data operators call "operational definitions" which clearly defines the measure, the instrument to measure and the procedure for measuring. A good quality indicator has a well written and well defined explanation that has been agreed upon by all the stakeholders. In quality, the indicator is spelled out on an Indicator Specification Sheet (ISS). Indicator Specification Sheet should have a section on it where the questions that the stakeholders are trying to answer is translated into a workable data sheet that give the data operator or specialist at a minimum - answers to all of the following data collection questions;

1. Who will collect the data?

2. Why are you collecting the data?

3. What methods will be used to collect it?

4. What specific data elements to be collected?

5. When will the data be collected?

6. Where will the data be collected?

7. How will the data be measured?

8. What format or medium will the data/measure be presented or reported?

9. What training is needed for the data collection?

The Concept of Reverse Engineering

Indicators also help to determine what a data system should look like prior to actually spending the money to develop one. The concept of reverse engineering is where a data system designer actually asks the questions to be answered by the data system **BEFORE** it is actually built - a rather novel concept which you would think should be widespread, but not so as I have learned. In many cases, data systems developed at enormous costs and the designing of such systems were primarily done by who else, but the data specialists and technical experts who had no idea what the system was really supposed to do.[20] [26] It's not their fault. Most of the time they built what the users wanted - a data system with little forethought as to the purpose of the data.

Consequently, EMS has many data systems today that produce information that often has little or no value to the end users. Indicators can work against this problem by being an integral part of the original design of a data system. By first asking the questions of stakeholders and end users, the answers can be defined and consensus can be reached as to the purpose of the data. Then once all the indicators are established, the data can now be determined and defined to produce the data. Hence, the concept of reverse or should it really be called "what we should have done to begin with?" engineering is born. How much money could have been saved by using indicators to develop data systems from the beginning?

THE DATA MACHINE

"If you build it, will they come?"

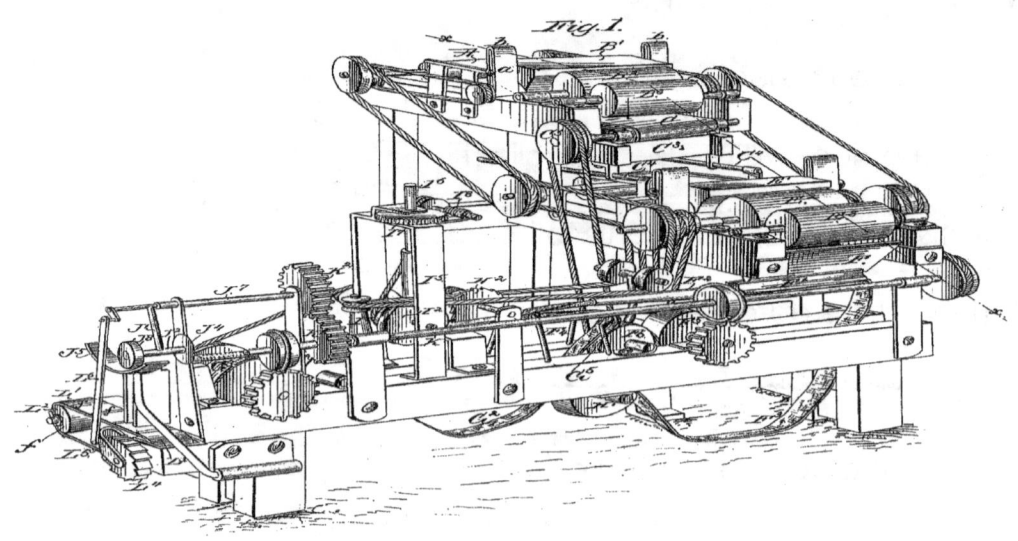

PART II
The Quality Indicator Defined

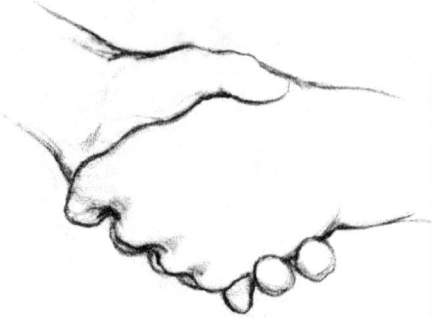

The true power of a quality indicator comes from those who gave birth to it and consensus is the cornerstone in the building of an indicator (8). One of the bigger mistakes made by Quality Managers is to collect and organize data into a report that gets presented to users who have never had a chance to define what it is they are now viewing and judging. On the other hand, if information is presented to the end users who have defined that information through agreement and now trust what they see in front of them, moving forward on evaluating performance is a much easier process.

Consensus is the foundation that supports all things quality. It is the glue that holds together all progress of any powerful and productive CQI program. Consensus is built upon trust and trust is built upon sharing common understandings, definitions and knowledge of the subject to be shared. In today's quality improvement programs and especially in EMS, one of the most effective ways for Quality Mangers to meet these needs is through standardized training and tools that are consistent across all lines and disciplines of service

I would advocate that today's EMS Quality Manager should be the person within an organization who can lead with strong communication and consensus building skills. Most importantly, the manager should be the expert in effectively reaching consensus amongst the rank and file of an organization. Quality Managers should also have a clear process in place which provides valuable and trusted information and stimulates productive discussions about how to develop and improve services.

Every program and program manager has its own unique situation, expectations and results. What is most important is that we are all trained in a common approach to our work. While we are all unique, our training, definitions, and approach to collecting, evaluating and acting on our quality information should be standardized and common to all. This standardization begins with consensus between all of us on what a quality indicator says and does.

Today's quality improvement models has moved forward to a process where aggregate data is now evaluated as a system and with well-defined quality indicators that are watchful of activity and that point the way to improvement. In most cases, we now look at the system for flaws and not problems within the individual person or provider. (11) (27)

The Quality Indicator as a Powerful Consensus Tool

In the world of quality improvement, indicators are your "go-to" tool for building consensus and trust of your information within a CQI constituent group. [19] An important objective in the CQI process is trying to eliminate as much controversy and mistrust as possible. This is not always an easy task considering the host of aggressive personalities that EMS tends to attract as a profession. It is often said in quality circles that "he who has the data is king" and I strongly agree. But there are conditions to my agreement. First, it is critical that all the data is collected in a way and from a source that has been previously agreed upon by the group. If this condition is satisfied and the data is considered to be trustworthy by the group, then I have seen with my own eyes the almost complete elimination of subjective controversy and innuendo that can be slung around a room from one person to another without regard to what is the truth. The nice thing is we're pretty good at collecting data and throwing the money at it. The problem we often run into is even with good data we sometimes don't know how to communicate it to the group. This is where quality indicators become so important to the CQI process.

Organizing the data in a pre-determined and agreed upon format (quality indicators) takes away a lot of the problems inherent to a CQI group decision making process. While it seems to be impossible to eliminate controversy completely from a process, using indicators to show the data puts the information in a very objective format and tends to remove subjectivity, barriers and controversy. Quality indicators are the core method for communicating your data and should be the core tools of any EMS quality improvement program.

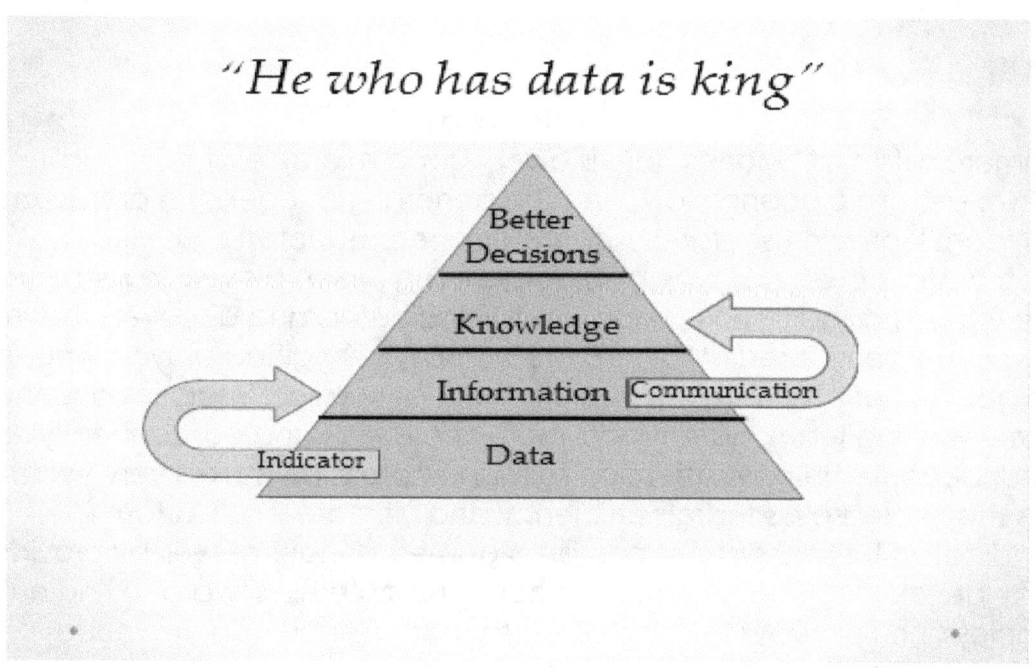

Consensus in Decision Making

Organizing and clearly communicating important information about data is the key to facilitating a good decision on the part of the users. Quality indicators are used to interpret information and help make decisions. As previously discussed, quality indicators are only a tool. People make decisions, not data and not indicators. An indicator helps a group of people to look at information and interpret what it means, and/or to decide if the subject of the indicator requires something to be done to make it better. Without the people, the quality indicator has no value and no meaning; on the other hand, a quality indicator is built and lives off of those who gave it birth and defined it. Evaluation is a process. Deciding what's important and what can make it better can be difficult if you are not organized in the approach.

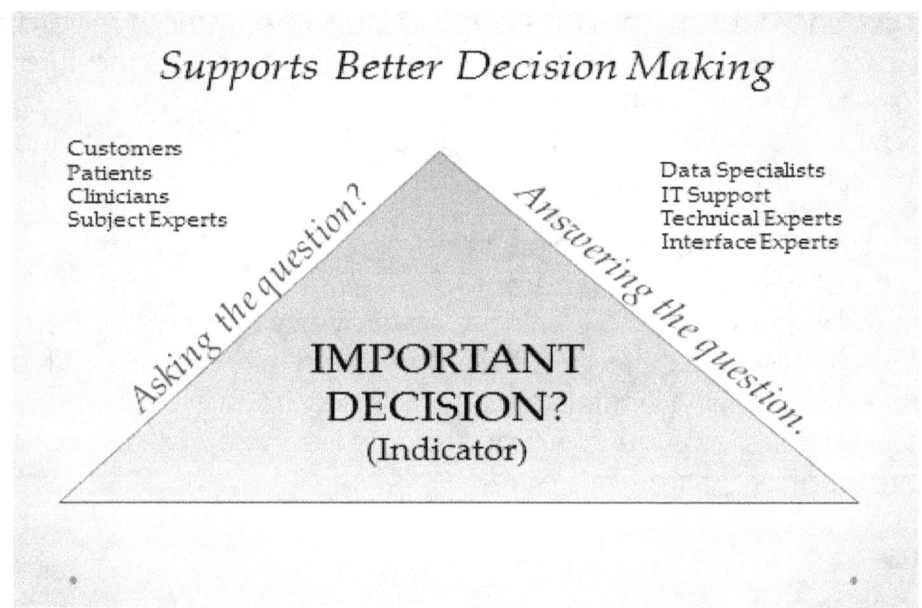

Supports Better Decision Making

Customers
Patients
Clinicians
Subject Experts

Asking the question?

Answering the question.

Data Specialists
IT Support
Technical Experts
Interface Experts

IMPORTANT DECISION?
(Indicator)

Money Ball

The commercial film hit "Money Ball" is a very good example of how quality indicators can save or generate economic value. The general manager of a professional baseball team learns to use statistics to determine productivity. He does not give reputation or star power any weight in determining which players to recruit to his team. He focuses primarily on obscure quality indicators and discovers that many players who are considered mediocre are actually very gifted players who can help his team get "out of their funk". He recruits them at mediocre salaries and then becomes a winning team that attracts many more fans and consequently revenues. In the end, because he pays attention to his indicators, he makes very valuable decisions that increase his team's efficiency and ultimately his bottom line. Quality indicators for EMS systems can be a game changer as well by providing a vehicle for developing consensus which can push systems forward to ring out inefficiencies and find ways to improve performance. Increasing revenues or saving costs is often a byproduct of a good quality process.

Quality Indicators vs. Scientific and Research Based Indicators

It's important not to get our concepts crossed up. Quality indicators strive to provide valuable and real time information; however, it is NOT held to the same rigors and discipline of scientific research. [19] CQI and the use of quality indicators can be better described as "soft science" that tends to provide a basis for change. The importance of and the difference is that indicators and CQI information should come from the people or organizations that generate the data and they should trust what we have put together. Another important point to those utilizing quality indicators is that "close does count". Quality indicators are not meant to be completely accurate, but to err on the side of false positives. As opposed to the rigors of science where accuracy and precision are required to reach conclusions, in quality there may be times indeed when having a good idea of where things are may suffice enough to take action. In other words, close counts in CQI.

When dealing with quality issues, sometimes close is good enough!

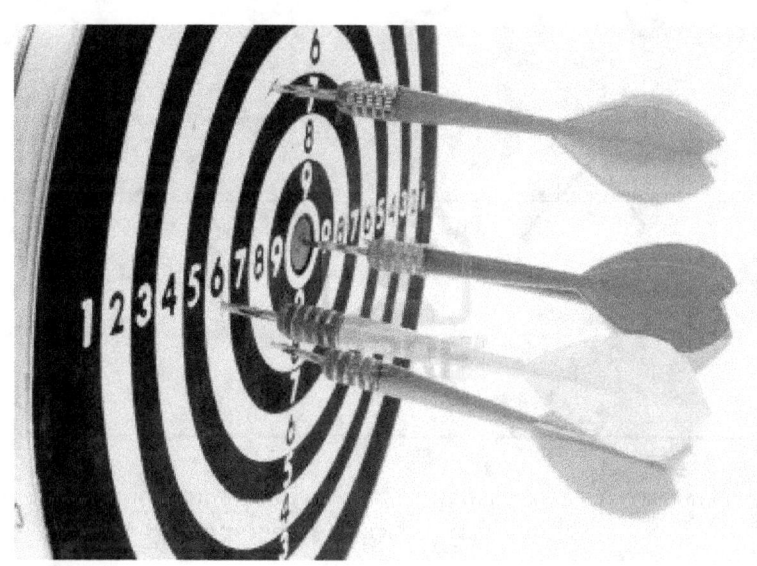

What are Quality Indicators?

Quality indicators are the tools that define the data, communicate the information, establish the consensus, stimulate the discussion and ultimately provide the proof that something is indeed better. In other words, CQI is heavily dependent on motivating people to be better just like the coaches of a sports team, quality indicators are the key tools that coaches use to motivate change and improvement.

It makes no difference what EMS culture you work within, whether a hospital, or the rank and file of a fire department, or in the management structure of a patient transportation industry or whether you choose traditional PDCA, Six Sigma, Lean, or Rapid Cycle Improvement as your model for CQI. It all comes down to communication and motivation and it is the quality indicator that provides the primary tool and language for accomplishing this ultimate goal. Quality Indicators are the guts of any well performing CQI program. The following are examples of actual EMS Quality Indicators in reporting format:

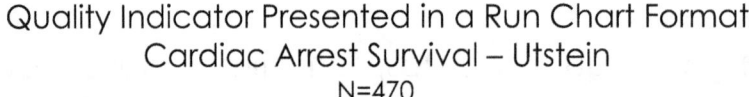

Quality Indicator Presented in a Run Chart Format
Cardiac Arrest Survival – Utstein
N=470

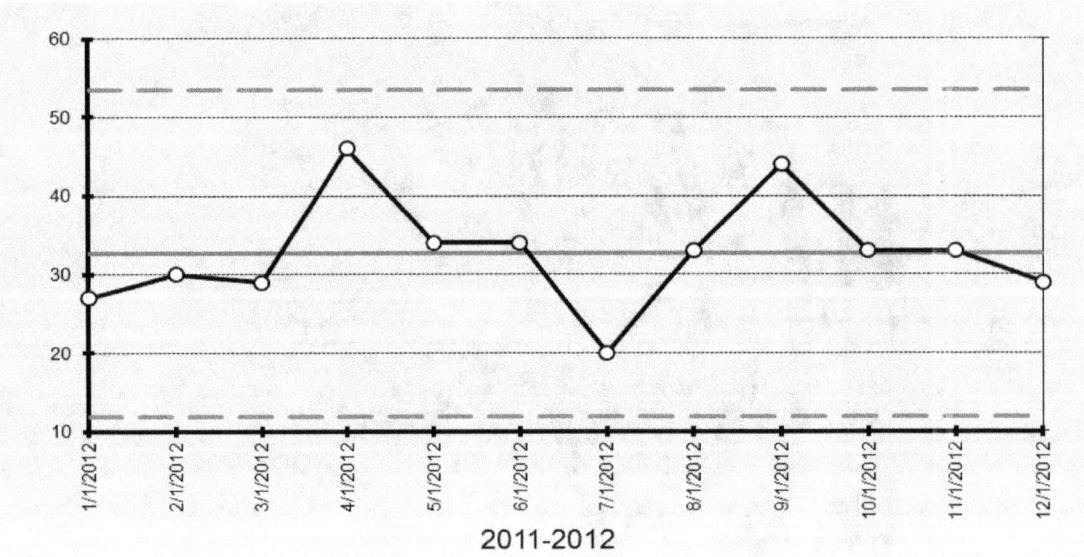

2011-2012

Examples of Actual EMS Quality Indicators
In Reporting Format

Actual EMS Quality Indicator Presented in a Pie Chart Format

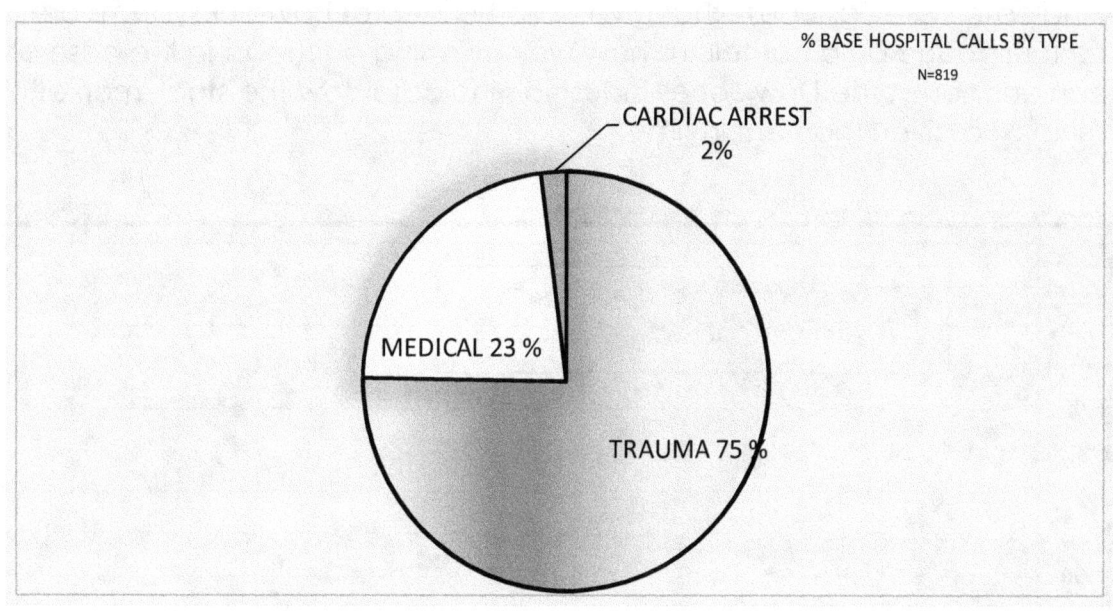

Actual EMS Quality Indicator Presented in a Column-Bar Chart Format

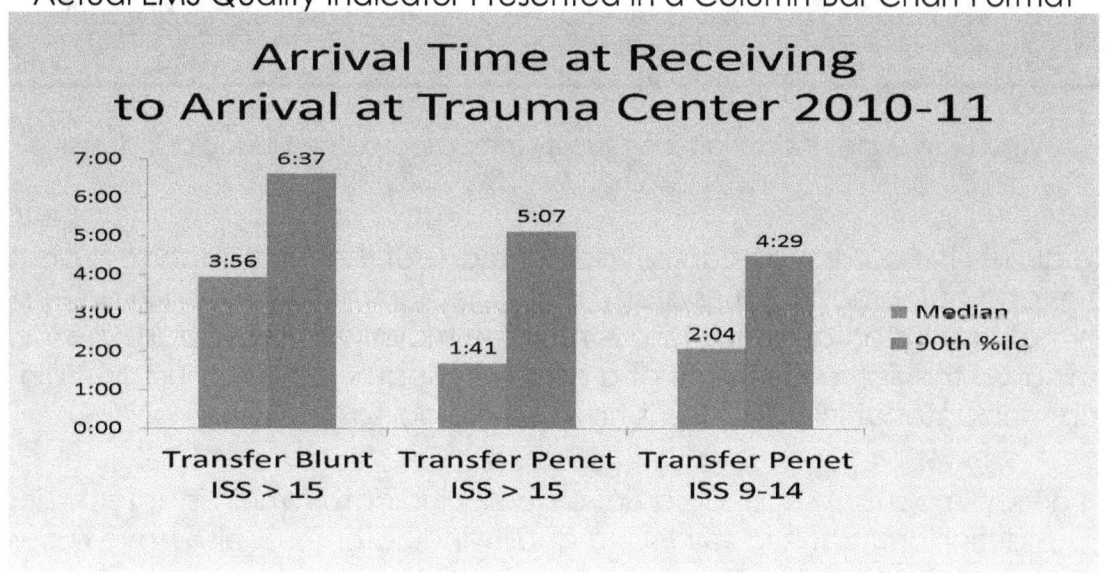

Quality Indicators are tools that are shaped and formed by those who use them. Often called quality measures, quality metrics, quality benchmarks, quality indicators can mean many things to many people. But for our purposes and in the simplest terms quality indicators are "gauges" that give us some idea of how our systems are doing. Just as a fuel gauge on a car tells us how we are doing on fuel or in the case of the American economy, the Dow Jones Industrials indicate how the stock market is performing at a given moment in time.

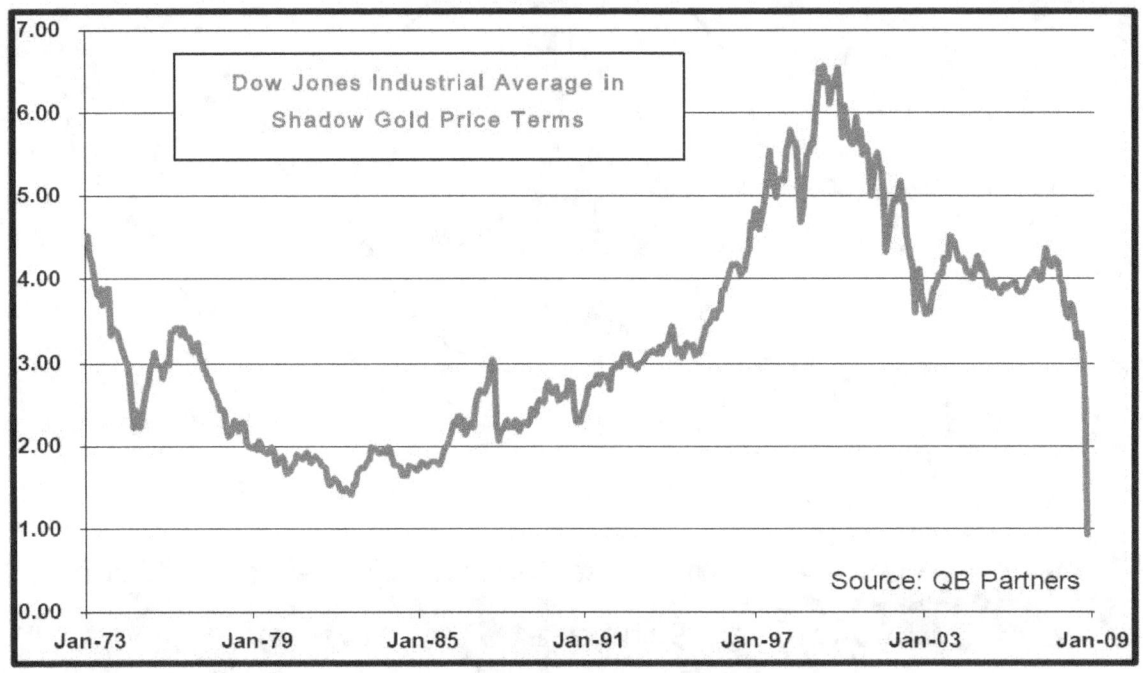

The Dow Jones Industrials is a Quality Indicator for the Financial Industry

A single quality indicator may contain one or many of the most important parts (activities and outcomes) of our system held together and displayed in an easy to read format that instantaneously tells us how the majority of these parts are performing. So the first requirement of a quality indicator is that it must contain value that communicates efficiently, "this is how we are doing". (16) (19) (20)

There is a very important second part of a quality indicator which is determining consensus definition. That is to say that a quality indicator must also have a generally accepted meaning that all the users trust and which says the same thing in the same way to all those who use it. In order for a quality indicator to function, it must have been previously defined and agreed to by its users. This is called consensus definition.

Just as when we measure the pulse of a patient whose rate is below 40 beats per minute (bpm), the pulse rate alone has little value to the clinician unless it can be put together with a patient that can be seen, touched and heard. In this case the indicator (pulse less than 40 bpm) must have a person for us to see so that we can define whether the rate is good or bad. In the case of a patient who is a triathlon athlete and who is fully alert with normal skin signs and in no apparent distress, this is perhaps a good pulse rate.

In much the same way, for us to truly understand and digest a quality indicator, we must define what it will mean first. An indicator must be defined prospectively by the users as to specifically what question will it answer and how the answer will be communicated. Therefore, it is paramount that all indicators start with a question that is agreed upon by all users through consensus. What do you want to know? How will it be answered? To answer these important definitions, the indicator needs to be captured and recorded on what we call an indicator specification sheet, or what is abbreviated as a "spec sheet" or "ISS".

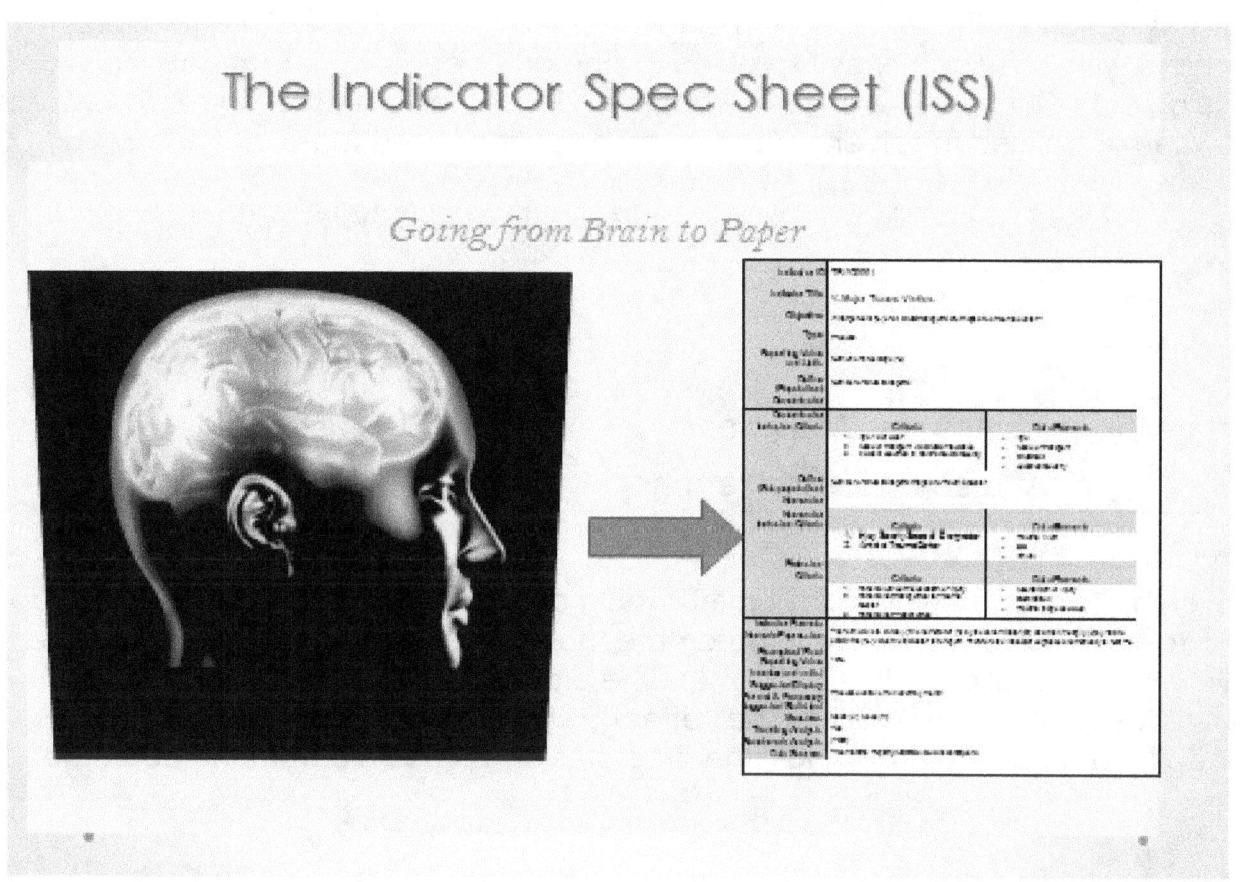

23

Structure, Process and Outcome

In most EMS systems, it is best to organize system information into three primary attributes (structure, process and outcome). (5) (6) (11)

The attributes-components of this system are expressed through quality indicators. These indicators are your tools for interpreting and communicating the need for change. This change is effected by pressures brought about by the collegial review and thoughtful decisions of the stakeholders within the system.

The change creates the pressures within the system to effect the change that hopefully in the end provides the inspired improvement in the outcome measures of our services in most cases. These attributes create the cause and the effect relationship within all quality systems, and accordingly apply as well and in the same way to the formal CQI circles where we EMS CQI managers live and breathe.

Together, these components make up the "great equation" that further defines the formal foundation for evaluating our systems by the use of quality indicators. For the purpose of illustration, we shall review the characteristics of the three types of quality attributes, which make up our system of evaluation, and also look at the relationship they have with one another as expressed in "the great equation". That equation is made up of the "things" in a system, what they do, or the "activities" within the system and when combined together, what outcomes do they produce?

EMS System Things + EMS System Activities = EMS System Effects

Structure + Process = Outcome		
Things + Activities	=	Results
AED's + Defibrillations	=	Survival

An even more specific way of saying this would be: People + Defibrillations = Cardiac Arrest Saves. In this case, the defibrillators are the "things" or structural attributes. The delivery of defibrillations is the "activity" or the process indicator and the cardiac arrest saves would be the result or the "effect". Therefore, we can then put this concept into CQI terms by saying: "the structures and process create the outcome."

24

Structural Indicators (Things)

Structural Indicators are things within a system, i.e. number of ambulances per patient population, number of hospitals with STEMI services, number of paramedics per response unit, number of trauma centers, etc. For example, there are 27 Advanced Life Support Units available to respond to emergencies in the EMS system.

Process Indicators (Activities)

These are activities or procedures that happen within a given system. For example; response times under eight minutes, proportion of cardiac arrest patients who receive defibrillations, IV starts, etc. Processes are often broken down into steps. For example, steps in the process of dispatching an ambulance would be: 1) 911 Call initiated; 2) 911 Call received; 3) Ambulance dispatched, etc.

Outcome Indicators (Effects)

By far the most important of the three types of indicators, outcome is where and what we are ultimately trying to improve. Outcome indicators are the actual results things have on the system based upon their respective activities or actions within the system. For example, it is a well-accepted theory that cardiac save rates (outcomes) are dependent upon the number of defibrillators (structures) available and how readily they are deployed (processes). One would conclude based upon solid science available in the literature, that the slower a EMS system responds with defibrillators to a cardiac arrest event, the lower the save rate and visa versa.

Other outcome measures would be: hospitals stay times, morbidity rates, mortality rates, etc. Obviously, the structures and processes in a system make up our "cause" in the analysis, while the outcome is the "effect". When we put it all together, we can see that the components are related to one another proportionally and can be expressed as an equation:

Structure (things) + Processes (activities) = Outcome (effect)

When we place numeric values to represent each of these components as illustrated above in our examples, we have transformed the components from an attribute to a quality indicator which can be quantified and qualified. Hence, it follows that these components are most often described numerically in the form of structure, process and outcome quality indicators. Using the indicator as our values, we call this expression the "great equation" because it clearly and concisely communicates both what and how we look at in our systems.

It tells the story that things are done in a system that have a cumulative effect and, like all great equations, one side directly affects the other. For example, by increasing the number of AEDs (structures) available in the system, we theoretically should improve the process (number of patients defibrillated) and that should have a cumulative-positive effect on the number of cardiac arrest survivors (outcomes).

The inverse is theoretically true as well. While all parts of the equation are important, a final point should be made about the proper interpretation of this equation. That is in all cases, we are most interested in making the outcome or the "end product" the primary focus of what we are really trying to improve. This is to say that while it is noble and most heartwarming to have an improved process such as increased intubation success rate, this attribute is meaningless if we are not improving the outcomes of those patients who need intubation in general.

Classifying EMS System Quality Indicators based upon Frequency of Use

Core, Tertiary and Adhoc Indicators
The use of quality indicators can be further organized and categorized by their particular importance and the frequency of their use within a system. The three major categories of indicators defined in this manner are: Core, Tertiary and Adhoc.

Core Indicators are chosen indicators within a system which tell a story of how well a system is doing overall at a glance. They are truly the "Dow Jones Industrials" of your EMS system. Just as the Dow Jones Industrials are the primary indicators of the New York Stock Exchange, Core Indicators within an EMS System should quickly answer the question, how is my system performing overall? In EMS systems, Core indicators tend to look at the most important primarily components such as cardiac arrest, trauma, stroke, base hospital, STEMI and system utilization. Core indicators such as those displayed below should be published regularly and should be open and available to the public to review and comment.

Example of an Actual Quality Indicator
Currently Being Used in a California EMS system.

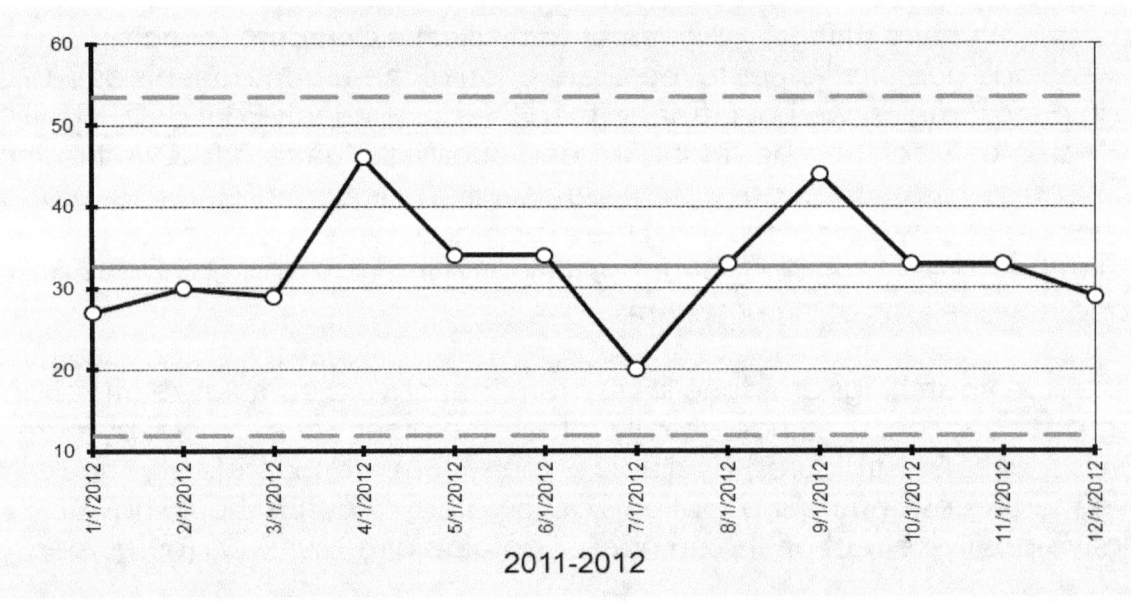

Cardiac Arrest Survival 2011 - AED

2011-2012

Tertiary Indicators are measures that should be at the fingertips because they indicate important performance information but do not necessarily need to be reported or published on a regular basis. Tertiary Indicators may be indicators that are looking more closely at a part or "component" of a core or outcome indicator. For example, save rates of an EMS System may be a core indicator and the time to defibrillation may be tertiary as well as a process which has an effect on the core.

Adhoc Indicators are indicators that are developed at will or at the discretion of the CQI program. They may be long term or short term. They may be structural, process, or outcome depending on objective. An example of Adhoc Indicators may be the development of an indicator that measures pediatric drug errors for a one year period. Once the information has been gathered, studied and acted upon, can then be discarded or used again as needed. Often Adhoc Indicators are used for special projects or immediate or temporary concerns of a CQI group regarding their system.

Bi-variable, Single-variable and Continuous-variable Indicators

Finally, indicators can also be classified by the way the data is collected and measured. For example, if the indicator end result is in percent (%), then that requires two pieces of data: first, the data for the numerator (small population) and then secondly, the data for the denominator (the larger population. Both of these portions of the data are required to perform the calculation to determine the final value of percent (%). One data value (numerator) is divided by the other value (denominator) to determine a percentage (%). Because we need **two values,** to get the final reporting value; this is called a **bi-variable** indicator.

If you were measuring only **one thing** such as the number of cars in a parking lot, then this would be a **single variable** indicator. There is no need for a numerator in a single-variable.

The third type is called a "**continuous**" variable which is where we are dealing with data from measurements that can **go on forever such as time, length,** etc. Because they are continuous, we usually put this type of data into a bell shaped curve and look to determine a percentile such as the 90th or 80th. Response time compliance is commonly reported this way. In this example, a continuous variable may be reported as the ambulance is on scene within 7 mins 90% of the time.

In the same way, different types of indicators require different types of indicator spec sheets to match up with the type of indicator we plan to develop. In EMS, we most often use a bi-variable and percent (%) as our reporting value. But when we are measuring things like response or on scene time then we like to use continuous and look at the 90th percentile as a standard. Accordingly, when we use a single variable, we are looking at just one thing and these are usually structural indicators such as the number of certified EMTs or number of ambulances.

Below are examples of blank bi-variable Indicator Spec Sheet (ISS)
Note: Blank ISS are available in the Resource Appendix at the back of this book.

BI-VARIABLE - INDICATOR SPECIFICATION SHEET

Measure Set	
Set Measure ID #	
Performance Measure Name	
Description	
Type of Measure	
Reporting Value	
Denominator Statement (population)	
Numerator Statement (sub-population)	
Indicator Formula Numeric Expression	
Example of Final Reporting Value	
Suggested Display Format & Frequency	
Suggested Statistical Measures	☐ Mean ☐ Median ☐ Variance ☐ Mode ☐ Standard Deviation
Trending Analysis	☐ Yes ☐ No
Benchmark Analysis	☐ Yes ☐ No
References	

DATA COLLECTION

Data Collection Approach	
Rationale for Data	
Sampling	☐ Yes ☐ No
Aggregation	☐ Yes ☐ No
Blinded	☐ Yes ☐ No
Minimum Data Values	30

DATA COLLECTION MATRIX

EMSA Core Measure ID: CAR-3									
DENOMINATOR Inclusion Criteria									
NEMSIS Element									
Field Value									
NUMERATOR Inclusion Criteria									
NEMSIS Element									
Field Value									
EXCLUSION Criteria									
NEMSIS Element									
Field Value									

PART III

Making a Quality Indicator

Quality Indicators can be developed by
Utilizing the following (3) three-step process;

- **Step # 1; The Indicator Specification Sheet (ISS)**; Developing an ISS involves engaging your stakeholders or subject expert group in asking the right questions about the right thing by the right people. This activity should result in the development of an ISS through consensus of the group. This step also requires the group to agree on where and how to get the data.

- **Step #2; Data Collection Matrix/Table:** This step begins with the review of the requested data identified in the top portion of the ISS. ITT and or data personnel should be involved at this point and should help to identify the specific data sources and elements necessary to complete the data collection & matrix portion of the ISS. The data is then queried and reported in a table or other standardized and acceptable format.

- **Step #3: Reporting Format or Chart:** The data table or report should be reviewed by members of the data team, Quality Manager, and the original core stakeholder group to validate the results. Once consensus is again met, the Quality Manager can then choose an appropriate reporting-display format and to convert the data to a display format most appropriate to the group.

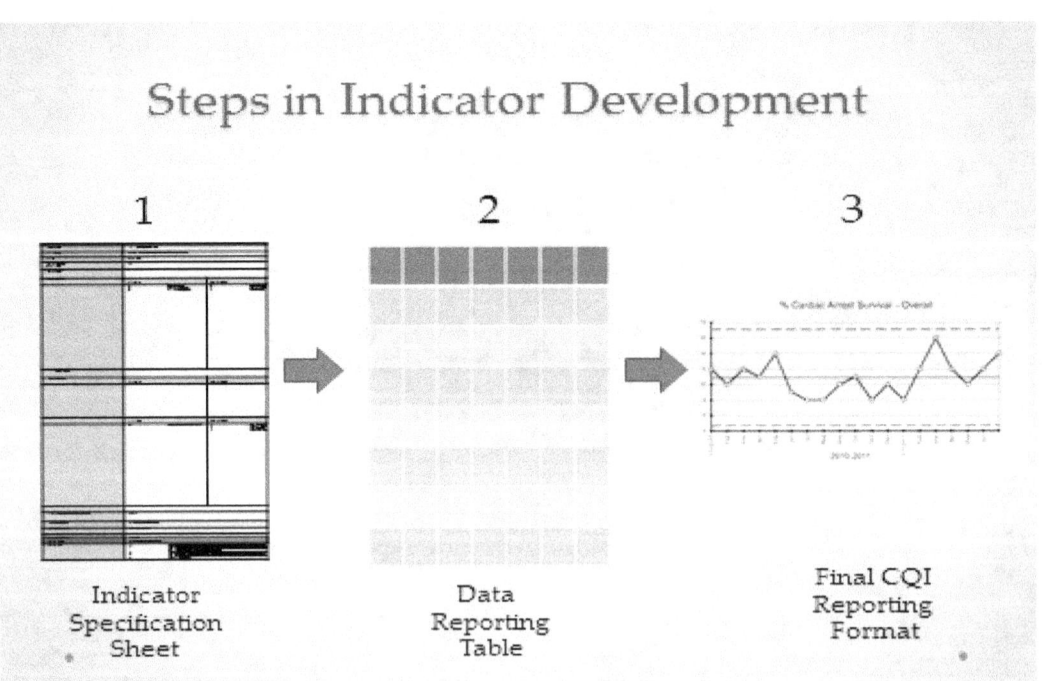

The following pages show an example of a fully completed Indicator Specification Sheet and a detailed step by step process for following the recommended three steps of indicator development.

BI-VARIABLE INDICATOR SPECIFICATION SHEET-EXAMPLE

Measure Set	Cardiac Arrest
Set Measure ID #	CAR-4
Performance Measure Name	% Out-of-Hospital Cardiac Arrests Survival to Hospital Discharge
Description	What is the percent (%) of patients who experience cardiac arrest of cardiac origin after the arrival of EMS providers that survive to be discharged from the hospital over a specific period of time?
Type of Measure	Outcome
Reporting Value	% Percentage
Denominator Statement (population)	Total number of patients experiencing cardiac arrest of cardiac origin after the arrival of EMS providers over a specified period of time
Numerator Statement (sub-population)	Total number of patients experiencing cardiac arrest of cardiac origin after the arrival of EMS providers that survive to discharge from the hospital over a specified period
Indicator Formula Numeric Expression	The formula is to divide (/) the numerator (N) by the denominator (D) and then multiply (x) by 100 to obtain the (%) value the indicator is to report. Therefore the indicator expressed numerically is N/D =%
Example Reporting Value	36%
Suggested Display Format & Frequency	Bar Chart; Run Chart
Suggested Statistical Measures	☐ Mean ■ Median ☐ Variance ☐ Mode ☐ Standard Deviation
Trending Analysis	■ Yes ☐ No
Benchmark Analysis	■ Yes ☐ No
References	

DATA COLLECTION	
Data Collection Approach	Retrospective data sources for required data elements include administrative data and pre-hospital care records. Variation may exist in the assignment of Chief Complaint coding; therefore, coding practices may require evaluation to ensure consistency.
Rationale for data collection	Cardiac Arrest survival has been shown to increase with early CPR and Automated External Defibrillation
Sampling	☐ Yes ■ No
Aggregation	■ Yes ☐ No
Blinded	☐ Yes ■ No
Minimum Data Values	30

DATA COLLECTION MATRIX

EMSA Core Measure ID: CAR-3	% Out-of-Hospital Cardiac Arrests Survival to Hospital Discharge									
DENOMINATOR Inclusion Criteria	Date of call	Card Arrest	Card Etiolog	EMS Arrival	Resus Attemp	Chest Comp	Vent Attemp	Defib Attemp		
NEMSIS Element	E05_10	E11_01	E11_02	E11_01	E11_03	E11_03	E11_03	E11_03		
Field Value	EE17	2240	2250	2245	2280	2290	2285	2280		
NUMERATOR Inclusion Criteria	Admit Hosp	Admit ICU	Releas Hosp	Trans Hosp						
NEMSIS Element	E11_01	E11_01	E11_01	E11_01						
Field Value	5335	5340	5355	5360						

Following the Three (3) Developmental Steps

Step1. Developing an Indicator Specification Sheet (ISS)

The primary QI tool in the development of a standardized EMS Quality Indicator is the ISS Tool. A method for developing and using the ISS to measure EMS system performance is described as follows;

Asking the Questions

Gather all stakeholders together and begin by brainstorming questions about the system that the group would like answered. Clearly state the purpose of the brainstorming session. Take a turn, in sequence, around the entire group. Do not criticize or discuss any ideas. Record each question carefully. Distributing a survey can also facilitate this step. Clarify the brainstorming questions and make sure everyone understands all the items. Categorize the questions based upon related subject matter and/or discipline, Prioritize or rank the questions based upon the level of importance to stakeholders or customers. If possible, narrow the list of questions by eliminating any duplication or questions, which may be too complex or off limits, i.e. finances, working conditions, etc.

Defining the Answers

Begin by clearly stating the question to be answered. Stratify the question (break down) into steps identifying the structures (who, what, where) and the activities (how) which lead to the outcome that will be measured. Note: stratification may lead to several smaller measurements; i.e. structures and processes, which affect the outcome indicator that answers the questions more fully. The smaller indicators may be relevant and should be developed individually, but meanwhile keep focused on the big picture (question to be answered). Further, stratification can be accomplished by utilizing a process flow chart to identify how, when, or where an existing structure or process occurs.

Determining the Type of Variable your Indicator will Require

Bi-variable reporting reports a single attribute (%) or item (fraction) based upon two separate variables (numbers) related to each other – such as the number of paramedics per ambulance (2:1 Ratio) or the percent of patients that receive bystander CPR (35%)

Continuous variable reporting are reports that have an established minimum and maximum value and where the data values can fall anywhere in between. Generally, these reports have an established threshold or standard attached to them such as the 90th percentile. For example, a fire district may report its response indicator at the 90th percentile as 4 mins. Or in other words, the EMS response units arrive on scene of their assigned emergency within 4 mins of dispatch 90% of the time. In order to determine a threshold, the data would first need to be organized into a bell shape curve and then the 90th percentile determined to reach the reported number.

Even though these numbers are infinite, they have limits that have been set such as time where an hour is 1-60 seconds. However, in theory a single value between the two limits could be an infinite or any number.

Single variable indicators report on a single (one) item or attribute based upon a single number of that item such the number of apples in a basket or the number of ambulances in the county (20 ambulances}. In this case only a single population of data points would be sought and only a denominator and no numerator is required

An ISS should be completed to further standardize and define how the information on the indicator will be gathered, and defined. The ISS is first completed by the initial CQI team made up of primary stakeholders and subject experts who have been organized to address the issue.

Step 2: Querying the Data
This step may require meeting face to face with data expert team/people to determine details. The following parts of the ISS may need to be clarified so that the persons performing the data query have a clear understanding of the expectations and limitations which may occur. At a minimum, the following components of the ISS should be elaborated.

1. Objective:
2. Denominator: to include population and inclusion/exclusion criteria
3. Numerator: to include population and inclusion/exclusion criteria
4. Final Table Reporting value:

Step 3: Validation and Reporting the Data Results
Validation of the information you have received back from your data team based upon your ISS is the next step in this process. The data is received back as raw data and usually in a table format. This data should have review and input from at least one of the original quality group that helped to develop the ISS and with a representative of the data professional team that performed the query.

The data table should be compared to the original ISS for intent and meaning. Consensus should be reached on the validity and accuracy of the data. Questions such as "is the answer to what we asked?" or "does the data table match up to the ISS data requirements? "should be initially resolved. Once consensus is reached, the quality leader or facilitator should decide on the best format to present the data to the relevant groups.

Data Translation Matrix

Below is an example of a Data Translation Matrix (DTM) Form which is a tool developed to do an inventory of data elements required to answer a quality indicator. The tool is helpful particularly for data system operators who need to know specifically which data points or elements are needed to provide the query. The DTM is often included in an Indicator Specification Sheet (ISS). The Resource Appendix of this book, contains ISS with the DTM is included at the bottom of the Sheet.

	Indicator Specification Sheet																
	FW-01A	FW-01B	FW-01C	FW-01D	FW-02A	FW-02B	FW-03	FW-04	FW-05	FW-06	FW-07	FW-08	FW-09	FW-10	FW-11	FW-15	FW-16
Date of Call	✓	✓	✓	✓	✓	✓	✓	✓	✓	✓	✓	✓	✓	✓	✓		
FD On-scene					✓	✓									✓		
FD Time Unit Assigned															✓		
EAP On-scene					✓	✓				✓	✓	✓	✓	✓			
EAP Time Call Received																	
Response Priority					✓	✓									✓		
FD Staging (yes/no or time)					✓	✓									✓		
City					✓	✓	✓	✓	✓	✓	✓	✓	✓	✓			
Primary Impression	✓	✓	✓	✓													
Age	✓	✓	✓	✓					✓								
Ethnicity							✓										
Gender								✓									

PART IV

Reporting & Presenting Quality Indicators

Converting the Data Table to a Report

Once the raw data has been validated and reviewed by the group, the quality leader or facilitator should determine the best format and media for displaying or reporting the indicator data to the groups for evaluation and decision making. The resource appendix at the end of this book has several charts and graphing examples to choose from with a basic explanation of what type of display to use based upon the data and subject of the indicator. Some basic principles of choosing an appropriate format include the following:

Simplicity

Choosing a format that is simple and easy to understand is best. Remember, we are not trying to impress people with our skills, but the true objective is to get your information across to as many people as possible in as short a period with as little explanation as possible. It is best to begin by asking:

How much information needs to be displayed?
What is most crucial for the group to see?
What is the most appropriate format?
Should I include more complex measurements?
Do I need measures of central tendency? (mean mode, etc)
Do I need measures of dispersion? (variance/ standard deviation)
Do I need Process Control Charts?
Do I need to do trending analysis?
Do I need Common-Cause and Special-Cause Analysis?

Trust and Ownership

Having the original ISS available or attached to the final indicator report is valuable in that it clarifies and defines the details of what is being displayed. It also brings the evaluators back to the origin of their beginnings. This fosters ownership of the indicator, what it is saying and ultimately provides the trust you need to make the indicator as displayed most meaningful and consensus oriented.

Medium for Communicating Indicators

The final indicator report can be communicated to the group by whatever means (power-point, electronic screen or hard copy) is most appropriate to your resources and environment. What is important here is that the attitude of your group may be dependent upon how you present. For example, sharing a wall screen vs. individual hard copies may foster team work and collaboration. Recognize your group's personality and choose the most appropriate medium for your goals.

Reporting Results; General Rule of Thumb

Structures (things) - usually are best represented by bar or pie graphs
Processes (activities) - are almost always best to show over time in a line graph. My favorites are Process (I) Charts or Run Charts. Outcomes (end results) - work best usually in a bar or column graph. There are some exceptions, but for the most part these rules apply to most situations.

Choosing the Right Type of Chart

Knowing which chart or reporting format is most appropriate for your presentation or report is crucial. It reflects your knowledge of the subject and also effects how confident you are in communicating trust of the data to CQI groups. Below are the types of charts most appropriate to the way in which you want to present the indicator result. Please be advised that all charts should have the (N) number displaying the number of data points used to develop the chart and the central measurements or mean or median.

To Compare

What it means: You want to compare one set of values with another.
Examples: Transports vs. Non Transports of Patients with Reported Seizure
Recommended charts to compare results:

Bar Chart

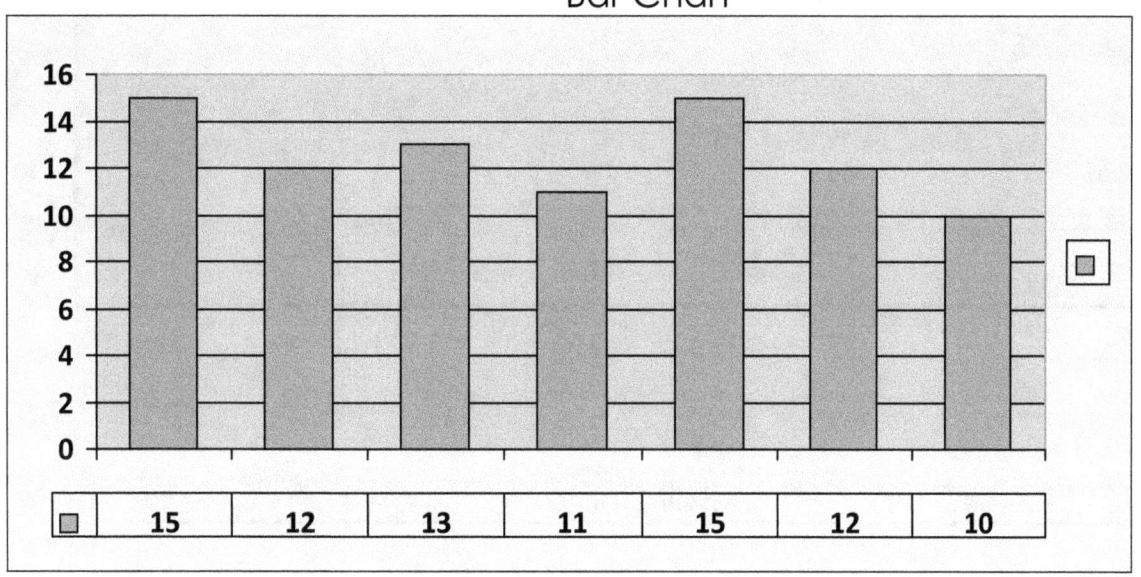

| | 15 | 12 | 13 | 11 | 15 | 12 | 10 |

Column Chart

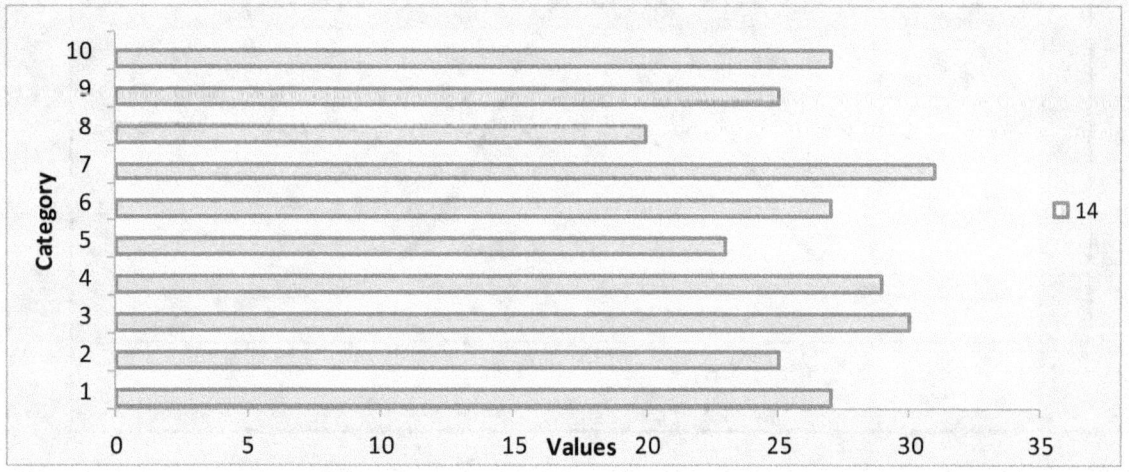

<u>To Show Distribution</u>
What it means: You want to show the distribution of a set of values to understand the outliers, normal ranges, etc. Recommended charts to show distribution of results:

Scatter Diagram

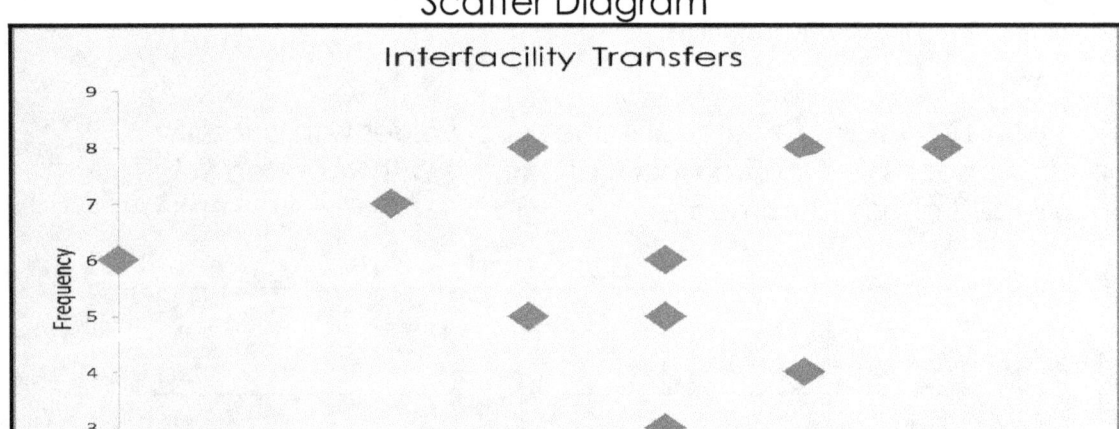

Bell Curve

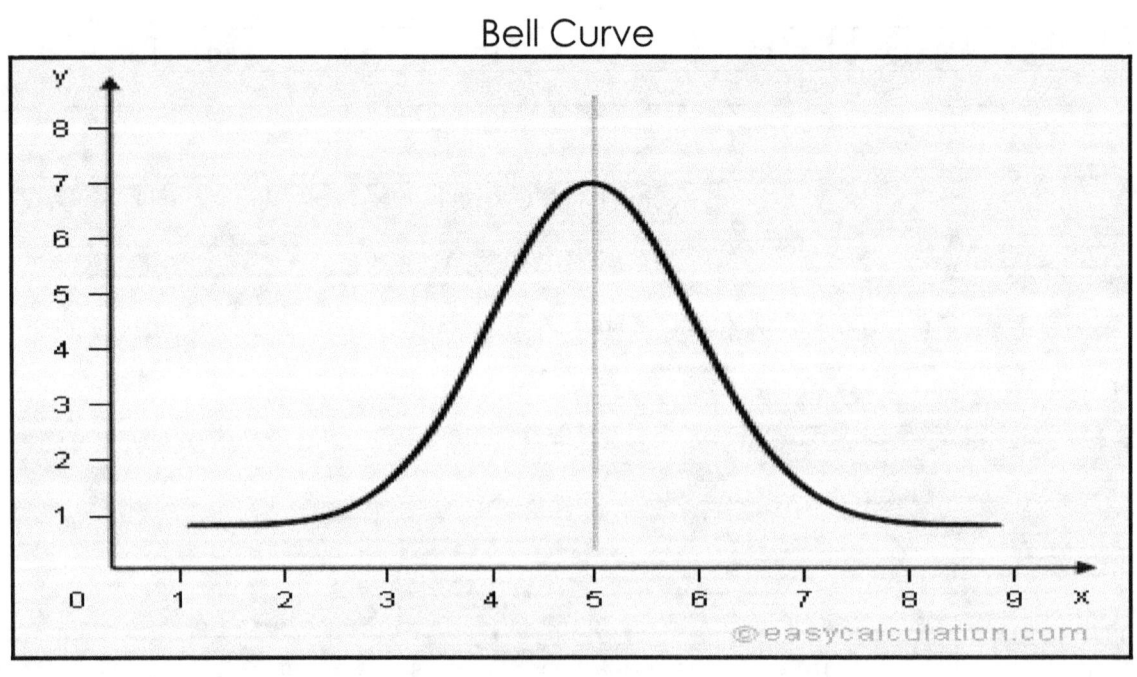

To Show Parts of a Whole (%)

When you want to show how various parts comprise the whole or how percentages (%) stack up. Recommended charts to show parts of a whole:

Pie Chart

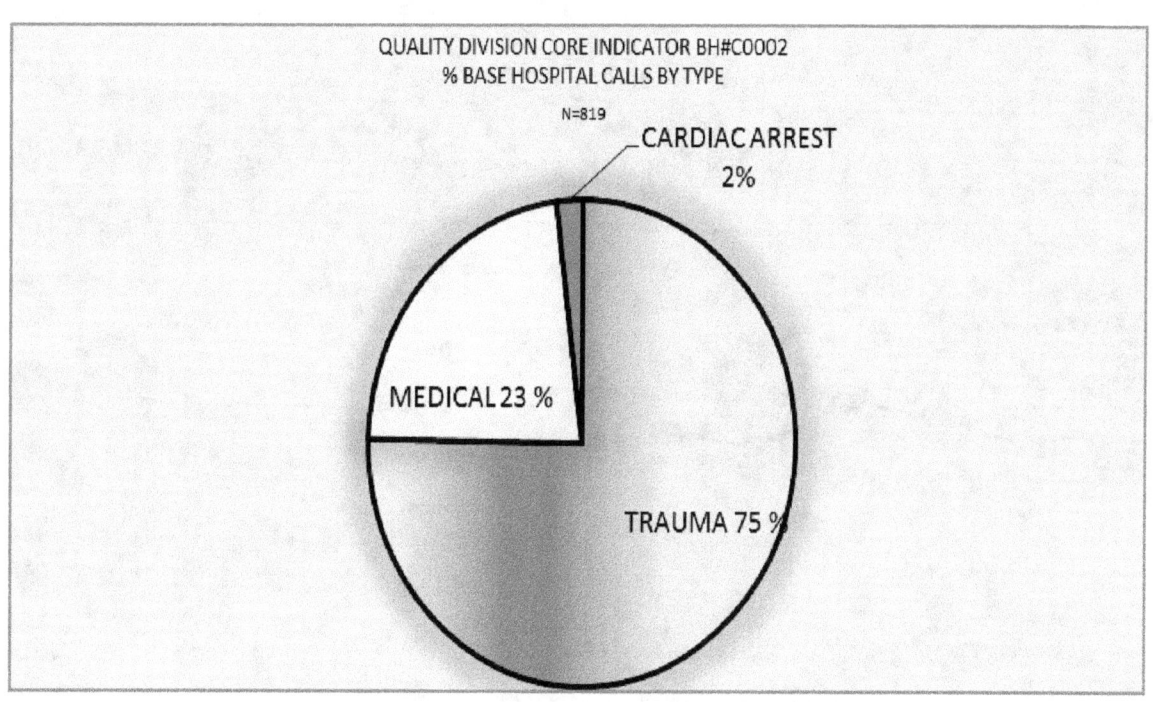

QUALITY DIVISION CORE INDICATOR BH#C0002
% BASE HOSPITAL CALLS BY TYPE

N=819

CARDIAC ARREST 2%

MEDICAL 23 %

TRAUMA 75 %

Histogram

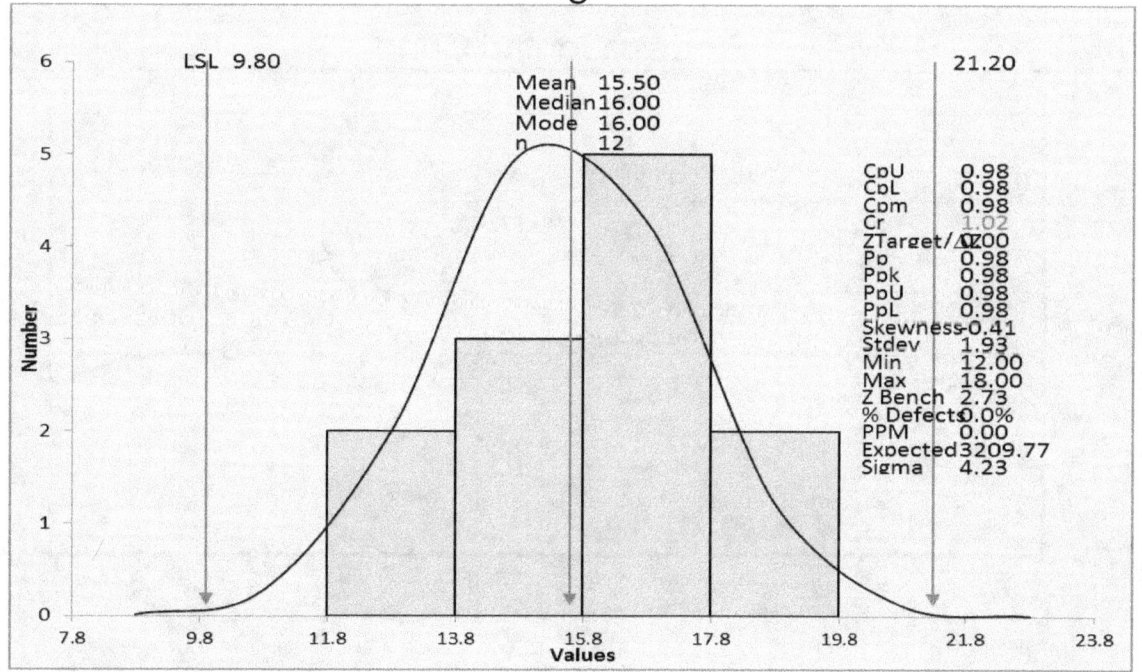

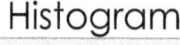

<u>To Show Deviations or Trend Over Time</u>

When you want to show how the data fluctuates or deviates (special cause) from the norm over specific periods of time. Recommended charts to show fluctuations, deviations, and trends:

Line Graph

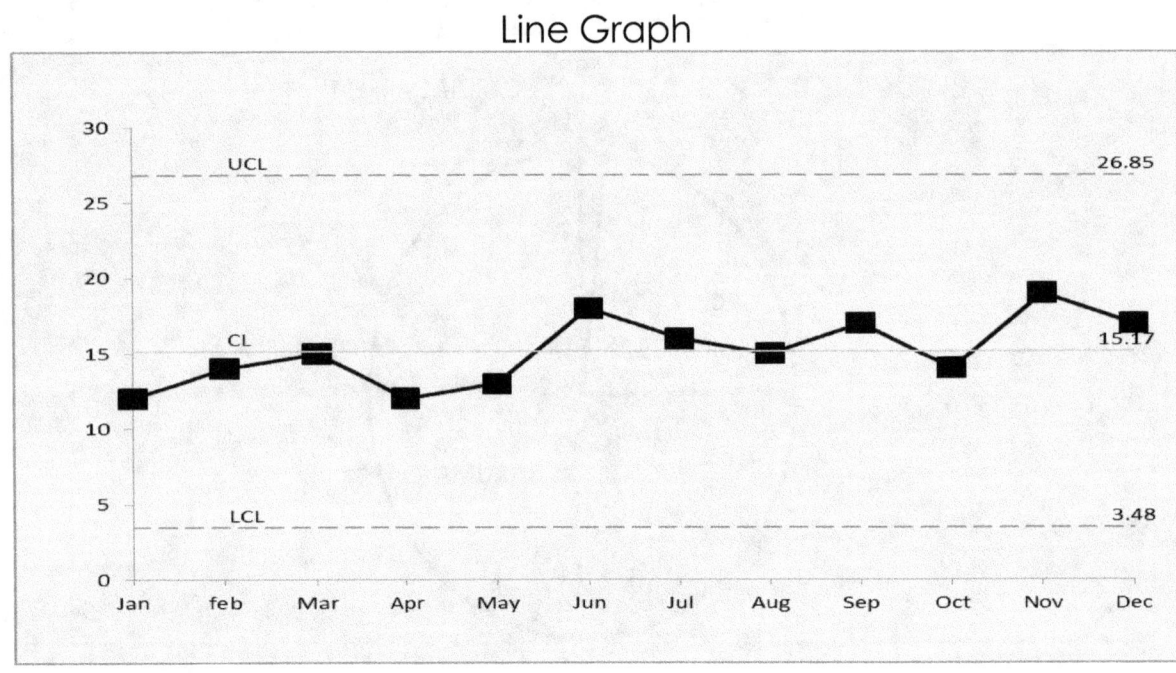

Process Control Chart

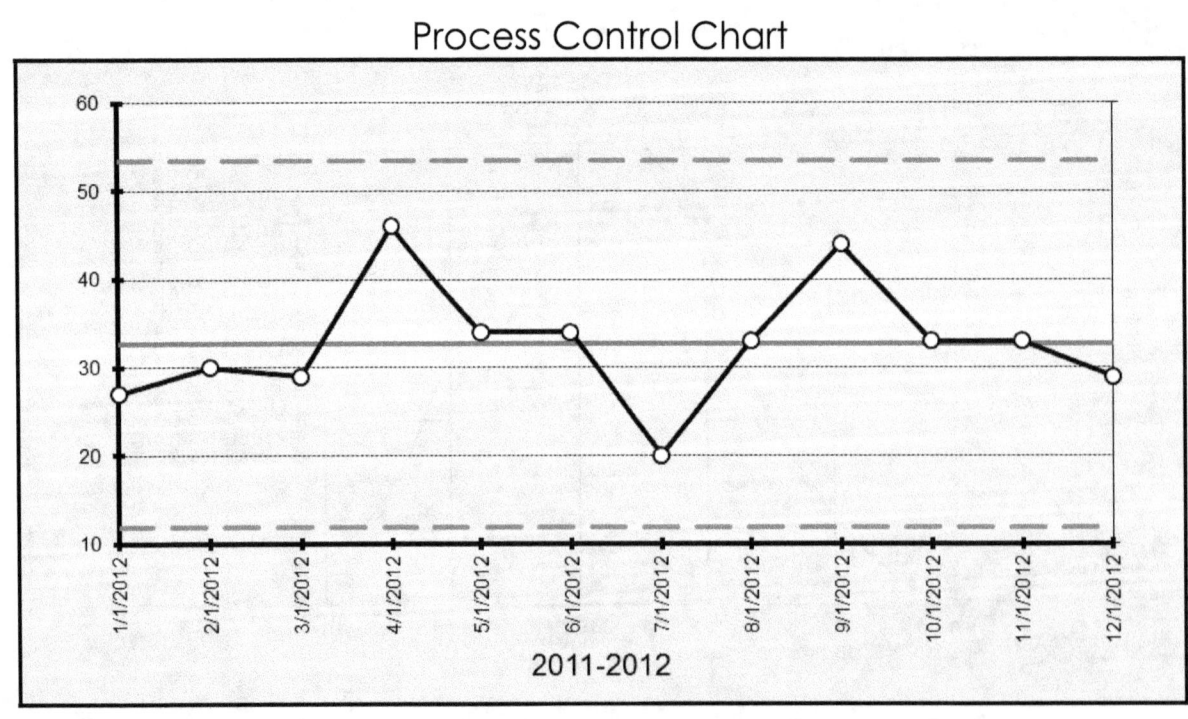

PART V

Evaluating Quality Indicators

Evaluating Your Quality Indicator

In EMS there are at a minimum, three (3) primary domains which drive the evaluation of what we do. (15) (21) (27) Those components are based upon patient safety, performance levels and costs of services. There are certainly many other points which can drive our EMS system, but for the most part these three domains seem to always be at the forefront of our day to day concerns;

The Three Domains

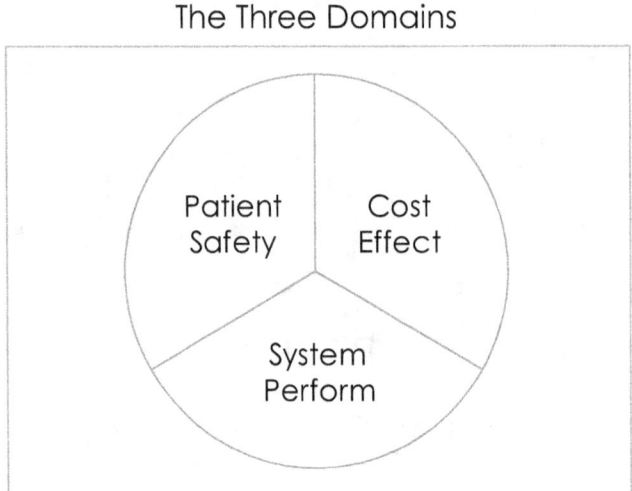

Accordingly, our evaluation of structures, processes and outcome indicators is guided by these subject domains and therefore suggests the following questions in evaluating a quality indicator in an EMS System. Is the activity or result safely in control? Could the performance level be better? Is it possible to reduce costs?

Four Step Evaluation Process

Facilitating an evaluation and a group decision regarding the results of a quality indicator can be challenging. Each quality leader should approach each group in the way and style which best suits the given purpose or goals of the group. A four (4) step process is proposed as a guideline for working through a quality indicator. The four steps are identified as; visualize, analyze, compromise, and actualize.

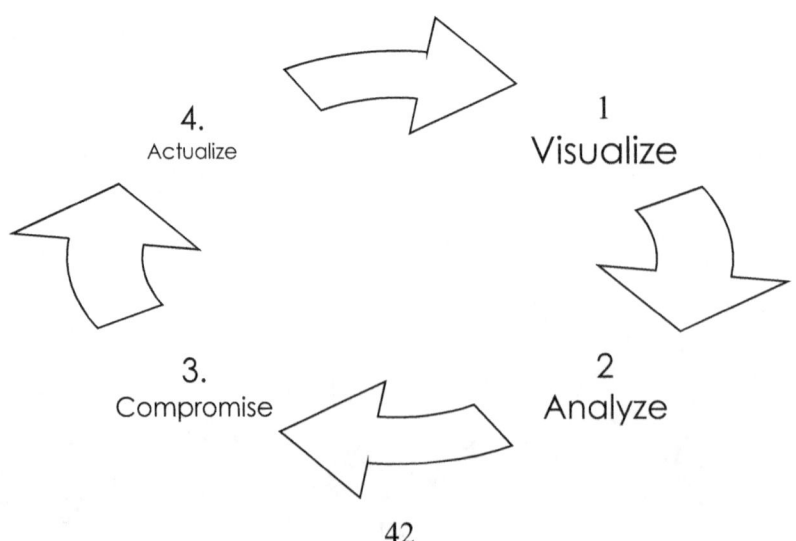

Step 1: Visualize

Choosing the appropriate display or reporting format is crucial to setting the stage for evaluation. The indicator as previously mentioned needs to be matched up with the most appropriate style of chart of graph. Making things simple and easy to comprehend builds trust and belief in the indicator. Please refer to Part IV of this book to review the appropriate format and type of chart to best demonstrate and communicate your indicator. The visual image should be as close to "self-explanatory" as possible. Make sure the image is complete to include the numbers used in the sample and the results of any statistical tests that were performed. When it comes to facilitating a decision process, there must first be a clear understanding on the expectation of the group deciding. In many cases a decision may not be required. An often used phrase in experienced CQI circles is that;

"The discussion may be more important than the outcome".

Secondly, information that is presented should be relevant, focused, concise, and in the simplest terms possible. Let's face it, everyone has enough work to do and you don't need to impress them with more work. They don't want to try and figure out what you are presenting. All indicators should be brought down to earth in their terminology and display format. Remember, simple is good. You will know quickly if your indicators are helpful and work based upon the response of you get from decisions makers. If they are focused and the discussion produces results, you win.

What's important? For a quality professional to facilitate a group looking at an indicator, the most important aspect is that the data before them must be trustworthy. Never bluff if you are not sure. Make sure all your information is true, accurate and it came from a trusted source which should be the very group that is looking at it. Choosing the most appropriate way to present the report is key to a successful evaluation process in any CQI program. For example, if the group is looking at a process or activity within a system such as the rate of medication administration errors over the last year, then it may be appropriate to show the information in the form of a process control chart showing activity plotted out over time. In this case, the control chart would provide an excellent visual showing both the level of performance and control in terms of what normally occurs.

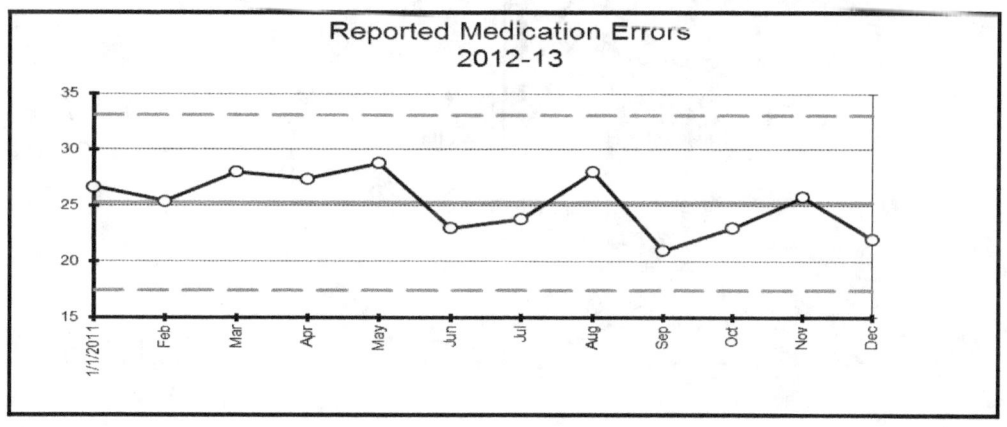

In contrast, if the group is interested only in an outcome indicator such a cardiac arrest survival rates, perhaps it is best evaluated by showing a bar chart which demonstrates differences from month to month or year to year.

% Cardiac Arrest Survival – Utstein

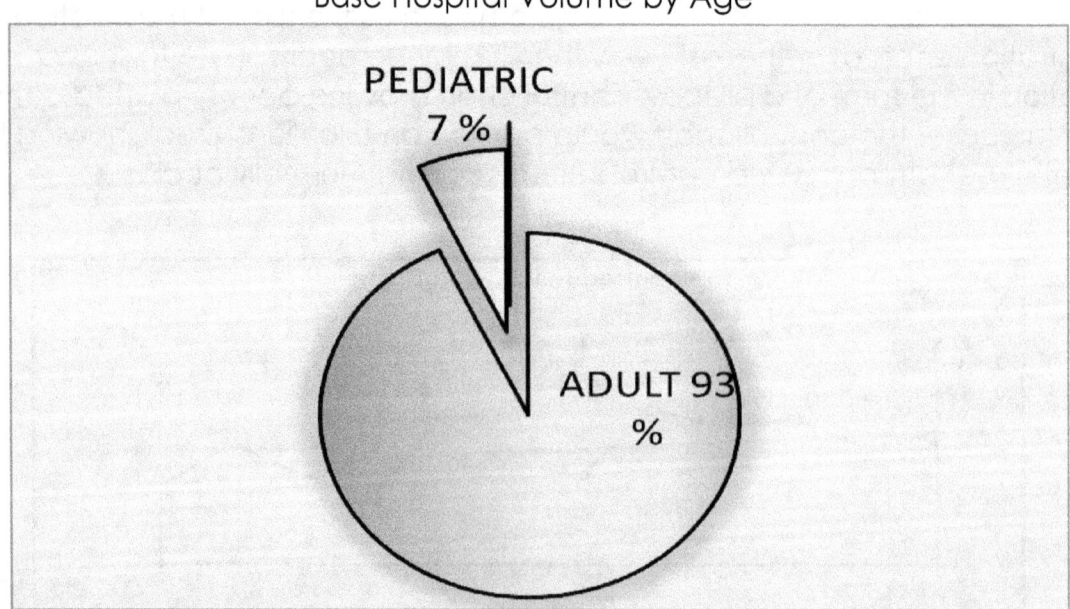

Thirdly, if the indicator is not complicated such as in the case of many structural indicators or when the indicator is asking what percent of something of the whole? Then a pie chart format may be best. Below is an example of a structural indicator shown in pie chart format and demonstrating the percentage of all trauma patients for a particular trauma center.

Base Hospital Volume by Age

Step 2: Analyze

In the next step, the indicator should be analyzed by the group for the following;

Collegial Review

It is not all that difficult to get people to offer an opinion on a particular subject. In the case of CQ indicator evaluation, this often remains true. However, in this case, it is the role of the facilitator to move the discussion along and to focus the group on what is objectively presented and what is "real" in terms of expectation. In facilitating the process it is important to once again remind the group that the data is theirs and the indicator was built by them through consensus. The main objective is to reach consensus based upon the four important questions.

1. Is the activity occurring in the EMS system safe?
2. Is the level of performance in the EMS system acceptable?
3. Can costs be reduced?
4. Can efficiencies be increased?

Safety

Data can be evaluated for safety by putting it into a process control chart to determine whether or not something has happened that may be a special cause, or in other words during the time the data was collected something "unsafe" may have happened. While the software programs perform many statistical tests, the primary focus of a control chart is to plot the data over time and look for any trends which may be out of control or unsafe. (17)

Process Variation

Process control charting programs are plentiful both in Excel and other formats. These programs are generally well developed and intuitive in their functional use for a CQI manager. For the most part, the EMS data is entered into an Excel spread sheet and then you push a button and the chart pops up. The software does all the statistical measurements and plots all the information in seconds. There are several software programs and vendors available to perform these operations. (2)

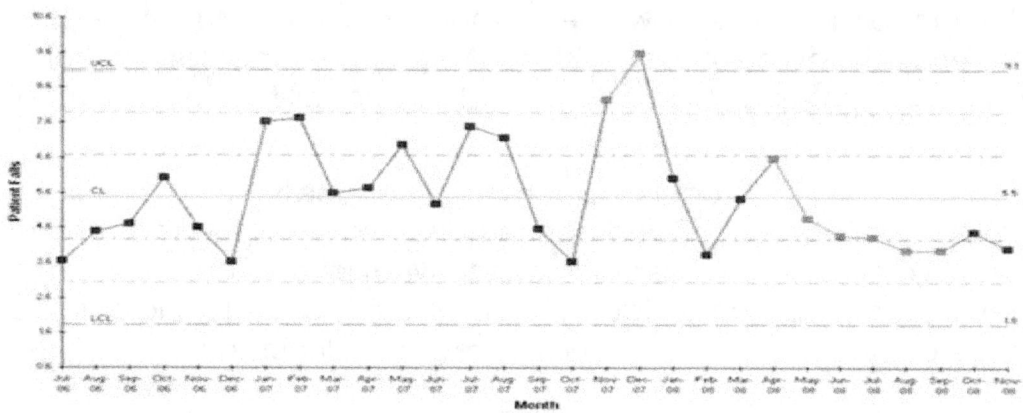

Control Chart in Excel

Evaluation of data by using graphic representations of activities
which show trends and variations over time

Common vs. Special Cause Variation

Each control chart is evaluated and analyzed for significant variation in activity. The two most common types of variation are termed "special and common". **Common cause** variation is characterized by predictability, irregularity and lack of significance in terms of values. **Special cause** is unanticipated, new, unpredictable, evidence of inherent change within a system. Special causation can be a serious signal that something has gone wrong in your system.

The first step in following up on a special cause flag is to check the data for an error. Most commonly special cause flags are the result of poorly defined indicators, poorly constructed data requests or queries. Checking to see if an error occurred along the way in collecting the data is by far the first step in addressing special cause. The next steps are to validate the special cause flag by stratification (drilling down) of the data to determine a root cause. Once the root cause is identified, then the new initiative to change or eliminate the cause to improve service can be isolated and addressed as a quality issue.

Performance Benchmarks

The second primary objective of evaluating an indicator is to reach a consensus on performance level. The question put forth to the evaluators is; does this performance meet our realistic expectations. In trying to determine "reasonable expectations", the use of benchmarks becomes helpful. Benchmarks are essentially historical gauges that someone else who was in the same situation as you already established and has been accepted as a legitimate level of care or quality.

Benchmarks should be based upon a similar or reasonably similar set of circumstances and they should be promulgated by people who have done the same thing under the same circumstance and moreover by people (peers) who on a collegial level have the same training and education. It is not always easy to find true benchmarks so often the group will find their own benchmarks (published studies, results, etc) that seem close enough and are acceptable to the group's expectations. Remember, this is quality improvement and not science. The standards are not as rigorous. (9) (27) (11)

Local or Community Standards

If there are no clear and established benchmarks available, then the community itself must decide in a collegial and gestalt manner, what level of care is acceptable to them as a standard. This can be facilitated by providing quality indicators of past performance of their own system for their review and discussion

Numbers are our Friends

Do we need to know statistics to use quality indicators? The quick and dirty answer is no. While Quality Indicators do contain statistical measures called measurements of central tendency and dispersion, it is not necessary for you to know how they were determined mathematically. For the most part, 99% of the time a computer program or statistician will have crunched the number for you. What is important is for you as a quality improvement professional to understand what the measurements mean. What are they measuring and why are they important? Simply put, a measurement of central tendency is exactly what it says, you are looking at the center (average) of a group of numbers and getting measurements of data based upon a bell shaped curve. These numbers are mean or median. Whereas measures of dispersion are also exactly as they are described, numbers that measure how far off (dispersed) the values are from the center or middle (mean)values. This is practically all you need to know. If things come up that require more mathematical prowess, then summon it. Let the "number crunchers" do their thing

Step 3: Compromise

Practical Consensus

Practical consensus is defined as reaching a group decision based upon the majority position as opposed to the unanimous position. This method often involves concessions on the part of some team members in that not all will agree on what they see and may interpret information differently. This is not always a conflict or a weakness, and perhaps in some cases it may be strength. Getting as many different views from as many different angles helps us all to see and understand things better. In many cases, listening to others interpretations and views is an education. But either the results are close enough that the majority is worth siding with or for the sake of teamwork or those that may not agree with an interpretation or decision may acquiesce for the sake of the team's progress. Perhaps moving ahead may well be in the end, the most correct and appropriate action.

Knowing When to Surrender

Forcing a decision can sometimes be the beginning of the end for a good quality improvement process. The underlying 'key" to any successful quality program is to have the motivation and a sense of ownership of the stakeholder group. Without these attributes, trust can easily be diminished and the entire project becomes futile. So sometimes it may be necessary to decide not to decide. This may be a case where in fact not doing anything is better than doing something. There is a saying that I often turn to when I am in this situation: "Never pass up an opportunity to keep your mouth shut." Sometimes it is better to leave something well alone. It may also be true that by doing nothing, you are likely doing the will of the group and saving future problems at the expense of not dealing with a single perceived problem.

The "Untouchables"

There will be times when after evaluating an indicator, the group is hopelessly deadlocked or ambiguous about whether action is required or not. In this case, the subject should be re-evaluated by the CQI facilitators to see if it can be more specific, or perhaps the subject is what could be termed an "untouchable." Untouchables are those subjects which deal with things not in our control such as collective bargaining Issues, fiscal budgetary issues, individual or non-system applications, and hidden agendas.

Highly controversial (political or fiscal) or emotional issues are very likely to end in divided responses, high levels of disagreement and may be almost impossible for practical consensus to be reached. In these severe cases, the issue may best be deferred to other routes and sources of resolution.

Step 4: Actualize

Once a quality indicator has been developed and defined by the stakeholders, it becomes the focal point for a group evaluation, interpretation and decision. Data is gathered based upon how the indicator defines it, and the information is put into a reporting format to be communicated (displayed) to the quality group (decision makers) so that a decision process can be made about it.

A decision is a commitment to a course of action that is intended to produce outcomes that are satisfying to the particular group of stakeholders. Whenever we involve people, we should involve the special skills of CQI trained personnel to again motivate, facilitate and promote consensus Reaching unanimous consensus is the ideal goal of the CQI decision making process.

The CQI facilitator should remain objective and be a non-voting member. In all cases, the decisions should be based upon all members present participating in a vote which can be formal or informal. There should be a clear end point where the decision regarding whether or not the activity or outcome is safe and performing satisfactorily, or that action to correct or improve, is warranted.

PART VI

Acting on Indicators
The Quality Initiative

The Action Plan
The Quality Initiative

Once a decision is reached, it should be recorded and archived. If the decision is that the performance is safe and acceptable, it should so be noted and archived into the meeting minutes. If the decision is to take action, a task team should be appointed by documenting the appointed members and leaders (see the resource appendix at the back of this document for an example of a task team improvement sheet).

Whatever approaches a group takes to improve a process, PDCA, Rapid Cycle, etc; the CQI Task team should have clear objectives for improvement and an improvement statement. See resource appendix for example of improvement statement which clearly identifies the goal of the task force and the objectives. The indicator should continue to be monitored and be readily available to the team at all times and through the entire improvement cycle.

Unfortunately, it has been my experience and is my current opinion that implementation is one of the "weaker" links in the chain of processes which make up a quality initiative. For the most part, we are pretty good at obtaining information and determining what isn't working well or as well as we would like it to work. We are even pretty good about deciding what to do about it.

But just like those of us who own lawns know, just because the length of the grass indicates we need to do something and we have a plan and the tools to do it, it isn't always easy to sustain the expectation of a well-manicured lawn. It takes energy and commitment (not to mention money) to make it happen. The following are some important points to assess when moving forward on an initiative.

Is there a grass roots commitment? Do you have the full backing of upper management and administration behind your project? This may be the time to stop and check on these two important steps in the implementation process. One of the ways to do this is to develop a specific action plan that defines the objectives of the project clearly and sets a specific but realistic timeline. These items should be presented to administrative oversight and to the working team once more for support and approval.

The following page contains an example of an action plan used to make the project specific and real. The action plan should clearly articulate the steps in the process, deadlines, expected outcomes and accountability.

ACTION PLAN SHEET

RCI

Action/Implementation Plan

RCI Project #   _____

RCI Project Name: _____

Implementation Statement and deadlines:

_____
_____
_____
_____

Action Steps: **Who? & by When?**

- ☐
- ☐
- ☐
- ☐
- ☐
- ☐
- ☐
- ☐
- ☐
- ☐
- ☐

Team Leader Name: _____

Team Facilitator Name: _____

Date: _____

Another distinctly important part of the "action" phase in the CQI process is to first check. It may be necessary to perform a functional or trial test before moving forward with a much larger or comprehensive implementation. Closing the Loop on questions or doubts the group may have identified, re-measuring to make sure your results are significant and keeping in touch with the original group as you proceed will all be steps which help to make the entire project real and legitimate. Making and revising indicators as you move along may become a core activity of the group facilitator.

Sustaining the Gain

Again, it is important to mention the importance of a tenacious follow up and sustainment plan. In many cases, I have seen this phase fall off on the gains simply because no one was paying attention. They were assuming the problem or improvement issue was simply over and done. This is why I consider the sustaining phase of a quality improvement program as possibly the "weakest" link in the entire process. The use of quality indicators is a vital component for keeping up with the difficult job of sustaining a successful quality initiative campaign. Simply because a project was successful and has been implemented, does not mean that it has been fully integrated into the culture and work force.

Continuous checking is important. Establishing "red flags" to tip quality personnel of relapses and signs that old habits are hard to fully break become as important as the original evaluation phase. In some ways, the sustaining phase of a quality project becomes even more valuable because all the effort and expense has taken place and we now simply just need to hold the line on the gain. The development or modification of quality indicators becomes important and should be developed in the same way, but now with timelines and milestones built into the measuring of long term improvement. Perhaps the indicator may now need to be classified as a core or tertiary indicator based upon the consensus of the quality leadership team.

Perhaps just as important is the organization's need to share the experience with others in the same or similar circumstance. The results of the project and the corresponding indicators should be shared with all who are stakeholders as well as those customers that may not be directly tied to your organization. One suggested way to accomplish this task is through transparency and the development of an Initiative Status Board which can be posted in plain view directly in the workplace. Below is an example of an Initiative Status Board.

2013-14 Quality Initiatives

PROJECT TITLE	OUTCOME STATEMENT	Phase I Staff Research & Review	Phase II Task Team QLC Review	Phase III Approval & Planning	Phase IV Implement	Phase V Monitoring	Phase VI Sustainability
Pre-Hospital "Push-Out" program	To increase the efficiency and verify implementation of system changes or improvement projects which are pushed out through our training	Staff is currently gathering data to see how well recent projects such a Ped med Safety and new Treatment Guidelines were pushed.	Action Plan -to be presented for approval at June 2013 meeting				
Pediatric Medication Safety	To reduce pediatric medication errors less than 1%	-Data received & reviewed by EMS Staff --Published in EMS Best Practices	Completed QLC review June 14, 2011. -Task team assigned and action planned approved	-New weight based measuring prototype and ped tx cards approved 7-2011, costs determined and ordered	Meeting 12/27, training session for distribution 12/28, All equipment and training distributed by	Staff to visit random stations to assure field personnel understand project objectives. Maintenance	Data to be collected and measured in the same way over the next six months will be evaluated at 6 month intervals.
Inter-Facility Transfers of Critical Trauma Patients	To significantly reduce the inter facility transfer times of critical trauma patients in CCC	- Data collected - Task Team to be appointed	Task team of local ED physicians and Trauma Center staff have had Adhoc meetings to develop	Team approved new transfer center at JMMC. Transfer center went into operation	Adhoc meeting to be scheduled in 2013 to check status		

Thinking outside the Box

Another often used statement that travels in many of the healthcare and affiliated quality circles which promotes this concept is to "steal shamelessly and share generously". This philosophy helps all to become better at what we do and in where we are going in our own plights. It is both very helpful and productive for us to help others improve because it allows the whole industry to be better.

As part of the implementation process in CQI, many program leaders often turn to training as both traditional and important component in changing behavior or improving skills as a form of total system improvement. I would like to challenge our leadership to find new and better ways to provide CQI training other than the traditional classroom format. The following are just some of the suggested ways to implement training for whatever improvement is in target.

Almost Real Time Training (ARTT)

Modeled after the mass casualty medical training programs, ARTT takes the training to the actual work location of the principle worker as he is performing the job. An example would be to actually call or radio in to a dispatcher and practice an exercise where a disaster has occurred and the dispatcher/trainee is acting out their new role and process for the plan.

Another is to have a sort of "tailgate" process where supervisors on duty perform actual practical training with the on-coming shifts as they arrive and perform their daily check outs on their units. Short and concise is the key to this learning process.

In both of these examples, the trainee is actually practicing in the real work environment and building memory and skills for when an actual event occurs. In the event that later they do use the new procedure or skill, they would then be in the same place where they were trained prior and thus they would have better recall and comfort level.

The Student Becomes the Teacher

This technique although not new is as simple as it sounds. Important concepts of the training become a curriculum of the student's development – "No better way to learn than to teach".

In this technique, end users are encourages and/or elect to be in leadership roles and to develop and create learning environments for their peers and fellow professionals. Moreover, they are placed in the role of "quasi" experts and this becomes a strong motivation for them to learn and understand the quality project or initiative being promoted by the organization.

Sharing the Wealth

In some cases, it may be good to provide the data and indicators used to forge decisions and action plans in the project or quality initiative. This action may serve to help the workers understand the value and logic of what they are doing. This goal can be done objectively sharing the information in a way that helps them trust what you are doing in your action plan.

Quality Improvement Stress Debriefing (QISD)

Following much of the same model for the well-known "CISD", this process is similar in that it consists of immediate defusing of complicated and extra-ordinary EMS events where positive constructive points of education can be facilitated and obtained. This may require a facilitator to lead the group in deciphering the step by steps actions that occurred at the scene of the event and then to develop consensus of the group in picking out the major learning points going forward. In this process, there is an emphasis on looking at the event from a system approach and not from an individual approach. There should also be an emphasis on learning and replacing what may have went wrong to what can be done in the future to make it right or better.

Putting It All Together
An Actual Case Study

A EMS System Goes Full Circle

How We Got Started

Ok, so how does this all work? The following is an illustration of the entire CQI process which begins with the identification of a potential issue to the development and evaluation of an Adhoc quality indicator within an organized EMS System. Although the project involves an actual process that has been documented and published, the project remains active and therefore for confidential reasons, the identification of the organization will remain concealed.

What Needed to Get Better

In February of 2011 we received the below Patient Safety Events Report via the EMS office fax. The event was evaluated and resolved to the satisfaction of Medical Director. However, the event was discussed at the Quality Leadership Committee (QLC) and an Adhoc quality indicator was commissioned and developed to monitor the frequency of these incidents and to evaluate trends.

EMS EVENT REPORT FORM

Instructions: Reporting is encouraged by all who encounter an actual or potential Patient event, system concern, or exemplary care delivered that may have had an impact on the quality of care or the prevention of a potential safety event occurring within the EMS system.

Patient Name: Baby Johnson

Date: 10-14-11

Incident/PCR#: 888999000

Time: 1430 hrs.

Initiated by (Paramedic John – Rescue Services):

Contact Info: Joyce Kensington

Receiving Facility: Memorial Hospital

Event Location: 1340 17th Street # 202 NY, NY

Others involved with the incident. Please include name and contact info:

Paramedic Williams, / Nurse Collins

Details of Event: (provide facts, observations, and statements.)

Under-dose of Epinephrine per local protocol.

Immediate efforts to resolve this issue: Discussed issue with EMT. Advise EMS via event reporting.

No untoward effect noted

Could this event cause an threat to public health and safety? 0 No   0 Yes Possibly...

If yes, contact your supervisor and the EMS Agency as soon as possible: 000-000-0000

The below Quality Indicator was developed by consensus of the QLC and then it was implemented to collect the data. The data was collected by data specialists based upon the specifications identified in the ISS.

The Quality Indicator Specification Sheet (ISS)

Indicator ID	QIP1- Skills #1Meds	
Indicator Name	Pediatric Medication Inaccuracies	
Objective	What is the number per month of inaccurate medication doses given to pediatric patients by EMS Providers in Contra-Costa County?	
Class	Adhoc	
Type	Process	
Reporting Value and Units	Number of events per month	
Time Period	22 months - Jan 2009 to Oct 2010	
Define Denominator	Pediatric patients that receive medications given by EMS providers	
Denominator Inclusion Criteria	Criteria	Data Elements
	1. Age under 15 years 2. Scene location in Contra Costa County 3. Medication administration performed	
Define Numerator	Pediatric patients that received doses of 25% or more over or 25% or more under the recommended dose per Contra Costa County Prehospital Care Manual	
Numerator Inclusion Criteria	Criteria	Data Elements
	1. Dose of med over by 25% or more 2. Dose of med under by 25% or more	
Exclusion Criteria	Criteria	Data Elements
	1. Trauma patients 2. Age over 15 years 3. Oxygen administration	
Indicator Formula Numeric Expression	N/D=Number per month	
Final Reporting Value (number) and Units	Number per month	
Suggested Display Format	By month - Process Control Chart; I Chart; Bar Chart	
Suggested Statistical Measures	Show median; Sigma for limits; trending tests	
Trending Analysis	All	
Minimum Data Values	30	
Data Source	NEMSIS	

How We Confirmed That We Needed To Get Better

After 12 months of data was queried and verified, it was organized into the below tables and charts and then presented to the QLC.

PEDIATRIC MED ERRORS
254 total pediatric patients cases were evaluated.
3.5% (9) of these patients received doses at least 25% above the recommended.
7.9% (20) of these patients received doses at least 25% below the recommended.
Almost 50% of the errors were Children under three years
90% of the errors occurred with use of midazolam, morphine and epinephrine

Frequency of Pediatric Medication Errors 2011-12

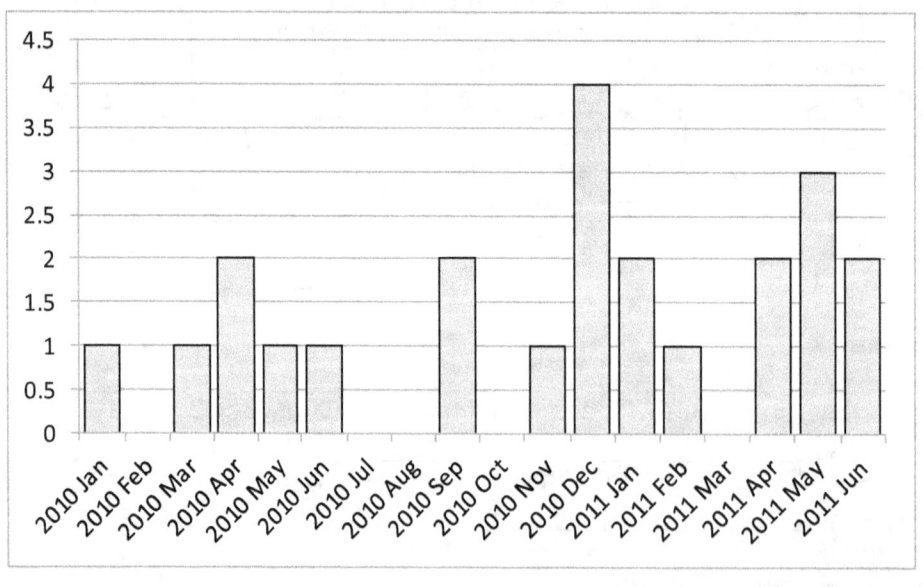

How We Reached Consensus
The Quality Leadership Council (QLC)

The charts were used to establish a common ground and were based upon data and benchmarks that were defined and agreed upon previously by the QLC. This helped to establish the trust when the indicator was later presented. There was very little controversy but considerable positive discussion about the results of the indicator query. It rapidly became clear to our medical directors and the members of the QLC that patient safety and performance needed to improve. Consensus was reached to move forward on appointing a smaller and more functional task team to further review the indicators and recommend an action plan to improve performance.

Below are actual minutes transcribed from the Quality Leadership Council.

Minutes from QLC meeting 9.14.11

Current CQI Projects	Discussion	Action
Ped Med Safety Initiative	On-going projects were discussed; • RCI Project - The patient safety events reporting system identified pediatric med errors as a potential issue. This incident will be addressed via the Rapid Cycle Improvement Process (RCI) and appointment of Task Team.. • Ped Med dose adjuncts were reviewed and discussed by the committee.	• The committee asked to be updated and report at next meeting on RCI project. • The committee requested to learn of any improvements or positive outcomes by next meeting

What We Did to Make It Better

A smaller and more functional task team met four times and worked out the following consensus action plan to improve performance. The plan called to improve the length based color coded pediatric tape and to make corresponding reference cards to effect an easier and more rapid determination of doses for pediatrics. In addition, on the job training was done with the providers actually using their own equipment at the back of their units. The training was followed by a short practical and dose calculation test. The following is the actual "action plan" as developed by the task team. The implementation/action process was completed in 60 days.

Action Plan: Rapid Cycle Improvement

RCI Project #   #762011

RCI Project Name: Pediatric Med Errors

Improvement Statement:

"Reduce the number of annual field pediatric medication errors to none (0) for a minimum of eighteen (18) consecutive months."

Objectives:

- To implement new tool (color coded tape and county approved matching pedi medication "quick reference cards) to determine and confirm the 5 rights of the pediatric patients.
- To make pedi-med reference tool available on both adult paramedic jump bags and in the shelves of the response units.
- Provide and communicate a clear mechanism for personnel to replace their field handbook when lost or damaged.
- Verbalize to confirm the dose and "how you got there" as a step in the administration of medications to all pedi-patients.
- Follow implementation of above changes with in-house training component.
- Put the word out that we are increasing our patient safety awareness with pediatric drug dosing.

Transparency & Dispersing of Information

Information regarding the performance and action planning of the Pediatric Medications Initiative were published in the system circular and also as part of the project status board posted at the EMS agency.

The following is the article from local EMS circular:

In EMS, safety is one of the cornerstones of our practice. Patient safety has become an overriding concern in the medical world, rightfully so because more than one million patients are harmed by medical errors in the United States each year. While EMS contributes a small fraction of these cases, we administer potent medications and the potential for error exists. One area of intense interest is pediatric medication safety, and the creation of a "safety culture" surrounding all drug administration.

While pediatric patients are encountered every day in EMS, the number of these patients we treat with parenteral medications is quite small. In a recent study, medications given via IV, IM, IO or subcutaneous routes were administered to 254 pediatric patients in Contra Costa over 18 months, meaning around 14 cases per month or less than one case every other day.

Out of all patient contacts, less than 3 out of every 1000 are pediatric patients who receive a parenteral medication. Few items in the spectrum of EMS care are done less frequently. Given several hundred paramedics in our system, chances are slim that a paramedic will be faced with administering a parenteral drug to a child more than perhaps once or twice a year, and some providers may not give a drug for several years.

Out of those 254 patients, 9 patients (3.5%) received medication doses more than 25% higher than the recommended dose. Not surprisingly, all nine patients with high doses were under 3 years of age, as the margin for error is less in smaller children. Another 20 (7.9%) received doses more than 25% below the recommended dose. Nearly half of those errors were in children under 3.

A dosing error was made in one out of every nine cases. No major adverse reactions occurred in these patients, but 90% of the errors occurred with use of midazolam, morphine, and epinephrine, the most potent medications in our drug box. While excessive drug administration has the most serious potential for harm, low dosing can result in less effectiveness of pain and seizure control, and may also lead to less than optimal treatment of serious allergic reactions. Accurate dosing is crucial, and our practice clearly has room for improvement.

Creating a culture of safety means that our procedures to provide pediatric medications need to be straightforward and that each time a medication is given, safe practices are followed.

These safe practices include:

- Careful assessment of every patient to determine if a medication is indicated;

- Assessment of patient weight, either by length-based tape, patient or family history when available, and documentation of that weight in kg in the patient care record;

- Using reference materials in all cases to confirm dosing, both with respect to amount of drug, drug concentration, and route of administration. All drug charts are based on kg weight;

- Double-checking the intended dose of medication with another person on scene or with the base hospital;

- Careful documentation of the medication dose administered (documented in mg or g, not in ml or mg/kg).

These practices are intended to mirror the practices that hospitals have taken to improve safety. While some of our cases are urgent, a small period of time spent to verify dosage can be undertaken in the overwhelming majority of cases. Relying on memory for dosage or feeling the urgency to act without double-checking are behaviors that need to be extinguished.

Part of the approach to promoting pediatric medication safety is development of training and ongoing regular review of procedures necessary in all cases. Pediatric drug administration is an infrequent skill and it requires an approach that recognizes that paramedics encounter these situations rarely – therefore practice is necessary to maintain the skill and adherence to safety procedures.

Currently, an effort has been put forth to develop an outreach program for field providers and to see if we can engineer an even better process for assuring the safety of our pediatric population into the future.

Part of the action plan involved is getting approval and "buy in" from the administration as the CQI Task Team progressed. Below is a copy of a memo promoting CQI Task Team changes and requesting administrative approval.

MEMORANDUM

DATE: March 21, 2011

TO: EMS Director

FROM: EMS CQI Coordinator

SUBJECT: Pediatric Medication Dosage System

As you know, the EMS agency has recently worked with ALS providers to reduce the number of pediatric medication errors as part of a rapid cycle improvement program To address the action the team chose to reduce these errors, I am asking the agency to assist the task team by procuring the equipment chosen to reduce the errors.

The equipment consists of a length-weight based measuring tape which is color coded to weight much like the " -----------" version, but this tape is simplified and does not integrate the information directly on the tape. Instead, the tape works in collaboration with a laminated treatment system which has been pre-determined by local medical direction and which provides a good resource for off-line medical control because it can be updated annually.

The following is the logistics:

Units Required: (54) for deployment to active units and (6) for replacement as needed. (60) total units

Deployment: They would be deployed by ambulance provider through their Vehicle Service Technicians (VSTs).

**Maintenance and
Restock**:   The equipment would be inventoried and checked daily by on-going/off-going crews. Supervisors would be responsible for monitoring stock and delegating restock or resupply as needed through the VSTs.

Costs & Funding: The units currently list at $ 900 per unit. Total: $54,000.00
                        We may also be able to negotiate a lower price due to the volume of our needs.

The following are copies of skills exams executed at the job sites while providers were on-duty.

PEDIATRIC MED ADMIN
SKILLS EXAMINATION
SCENARIO #1

11 month old, 9 kg, male patient in mothers arms; 2nd and 3rd degree burns to left anterior chest and left upper arm circumferential. Total BSA burn approx. 30%. Burn due to hot water from pot boiling on stove; Pt. striped and placed supine on burn sheet.

PATIENT VITALS ARE STABLE: P-178; BP- radial pulse present and strong; R-36 non-labored, clear, full

Patient pain scale 9/10

TX: Oxygen via blow-by

Give appropriate pain medication;

Right patient?
Right drug?
Right dose?
Right route?
Right time?
Right reason:

PEDIATRIC MED ADMIN
SKILLS EXAMINATION
SCENARIO #2

6 kg infant with severe allergic reaction to skin cream. Pt. is decompensating
1st Give Epinephrine: 1 mg/kg = .06 ml of 1:1000 SC or IM
2nd Give Benadryl: 1 mg/kg = 6 mg or .12 ml

Right patient?
Right drug?
Right dose?
Right route?
Right time?
Right reason:

Twelve (12) Months Later - Promising Results

At the anniversary of the formal implementation of the Pediatric Medication Improvement Initiative, data was again collected based upon the original indicator specification sheet and placed in a chart to compare performance from then to now.

The following is the result of that second measure.

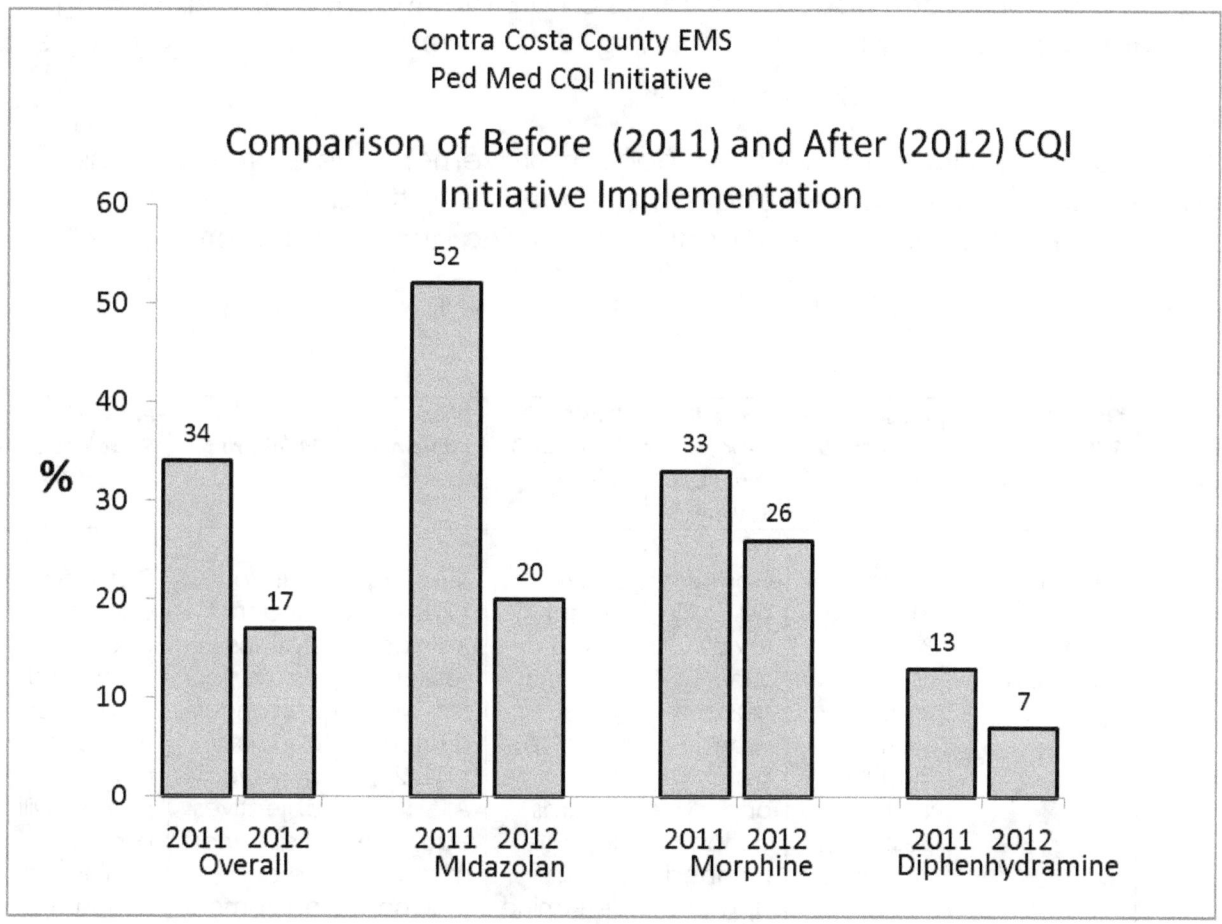

These results showed significant improvement and the QLC members were satisfied that performance had progressed. These results were posted and published out to the EMS system constituents. The QLC while pleased requested a strong sustainability program to maintain the gain and push forward for more performance improvement. The Task Team was re-assembled to implement and to establish checkpoints into the program and to establish a process where pediatric medication practices were reviewed annually by the QLC.

Pediatric Medication Initiative

Sustaining the Gain

Below is copy of the actual project status board for the Pediatric Medication Safety Initiative.

The initiative continues to be out in front of the organization visually as well as by placing the monitoring and update demands on a 6 month schedule for reporting. The sustainment plan mostly involves obtaining regular feedback to the QLC and field providers.

While the project continues to show very good improvement, there are concerns amongst members of the Quality Leadership Team and staff that a relapse may occur and so they continue to be diligent on collecting and reporting project status.

PROJECT TITLE	OUTCOME STATEMENT	Phase I Staff Research & Review	Phase II Task Team QLC Review	Phase III Approval & Planning	Phase IV Implement	Phase V Monitoring	Phase VI Sustainability
Pediatric Med Safety Initiative	To reduce pediatric medication errors less than 1%	-Data received & reviewed by EMS Staff -- Published in EMS Best Practices	Completed QLC review June 14, -Task team assigned and action planned approved July 8,11	-New weight based measuring prototype and ped tx cards approve, costs determined and ordered placed.	Meeting 12/27, training session for distribution 12/28, All equipment and training distributed by Implementation completed	Staff to visit random stations to assure field personnel understands project objectives. Maintenance and equipment replacement plan developed.	Data to be collected and measured in the same way over the next six months will be evaluated at 6 month intervals outcomes shared with community.

GLOSSARY OF TERMS

GLOSSARY OF TERMS

Action Plan – A written plan with objectives and steps to bring action with an organization to change or initiate an improvement in a process or outcome indicator.

Bar Chart - A graphic presentation which represents quantities through the use of bars of uniform width but heights proportional to number being represented.

Benchmarks: Known and accepted results. Quality measures of performance (structures, process, outcomes) often used synonymously with indicators, measures and metrics

Benchmarking - using known results of similar data measurements or tests as an impetus for achieving or surpassing a desired goal for improvement.

Best Practices - using the best known results of similar data

Beta Testing - To perform an exercise in obtaining and analyzing a specific indicator.

Bi-variable – indicator end result is in a reporting value that requires two sources of data.

Causation - the results of tests which are applied to a set of data points plotted on a process control chart. The tests determine whether or not a "special cause" exists within the data set and can explain unusual

CEMSIS - California Emergency Medical Services Information System.

Classification – Catalog titles given to indicators.

Continuous variable - indicator end result is in a reporting value that has infinite potential such as a measurement of time or length. Often measured by a benchmark potential such as the 90th percentile.

Control chart - Graphic presentation of a line graph specifically used to track the trend or performance of a process over time. Useful in demonstration process variability.

Core Indicator - The lead indicator being analyzed. Core indicators are composed of several sub-indicators (smaller indicators), which are major contributing factors to the final core indicator result.

Core Indicator Index # - Index number as classified by state EMS vision project.

Core Indicator name - Name given to the core indicator.

(D) Symbol - Represents denominator.

Data Aggregation - To blend all data together.

Data Blinded - Withholding identification of data sources or subjects.

Data Sampling - Obtaining information from a data source.

Data Linkage - Relating to two separate data sources or data banks to the same subject.

Data Stratification - Breaking down of the whole into smaller related sub-groups.

Denominator (D) Inclusion Criteria - Specific data element/points needed to perform the data query as related to the specific indicator.

Denominator (D) Data Source - The instrument used to capture the data.

Description of Indicator Formula – description of how indicator results are mathematically derived and determined.

Display Format - The medium or style in which the final indicator results are displayed

Domain of Performance - The category of performance being evaluated.

EMS Service Provider - An organization employing EMT-I, EMT-II, or EMT-P certified or licensed personnel for the delivery of emergency medical care to the sick and injured at the scene of an emergency and/or transport to a general acute care hospital.

EMS System Quality Improvement (EMS-QI) - An organized and formal effort to continually achieve superior outcomes through ongoing evaluation of performance indicators by system users and providers within an organized EMS Health Delivery System.

Effectiveness - How well a system is meeting an expressed objective or benchmark.

EQIP- EMS Quality Improvement Plan. A plan put together by an EMS service provider which details all aspects of their quality improvement activities.

Frequency – How often a system is meeting an expressed objective or benchmark.

Frequency of Display – How often a specific indicator unit should be displayed.

Histogram – A visual representation of the spread or distribution of the data categories.

GLOSSARY OF TERMS

Data are represented by bars of equal width or category and the height of these bars indicate the relative number of data points in each category.

Just In Time Training (JIT): A training style which emphasizes providing the training to the employee as they enter the working environment. Usually short and concise and done where the employee or worker would most likely be when the subject task would be done.

Indicator Specification Sheet (ISS) – A sheet of paper or electronic form which contains the standardized and accepted definitions and parameters for a quality indicator.

Indicator Formula Numeric Expression – Mathematical expression of how indicator result are determined and derived.

Indicator Reporting Value – The numeric value of the indicator result.

Lean – an established quality improvement program pioneered by the Toyota Corporation which focuses on work flows and cutting out waist.

Line graph – A visual display of data for comparison. Specific data points are entered by numbers are connected by a line. Useful in demonstrating a data pattern.

Linkage Options – The different elements that may be used to link two separate data sources or banks.

Metrics: Quality measures of performance (structures, process, and outcome). Term often used synonymously with indicators, measures and benchmarks.

Measures: Quality measures of performance (structures, process, and outcome) Term often used synonymously with indicators, measures and benchmarks.

Measures of central tendency – Values that describe the middle or majority of the data.

Measures of dispersion – Values that describe how the data is spread out from the average.

Mean – (Average) Sum of all data divided by the number of data points.

Median – The middle of all ranked and counted data points.

Minimum Data Values – The smallest number of data values which must be available to perform a measure and analysis.

Mode – The value repeated most often in the raw data.

(N) Symbol – Represents the numerator.

NEMSIS – National Emergency Medical Services Information System

Numerator (N) Data Source – The instrument used to capture the data.

Numerator (N) Inclusion Criteria – Specific data element/points needed to perform the data query as related to the specific indicator.

Objective – A description of the information that indicator is seeking to measure.

Outcome – The result of activities (processes) performed by attributes (structures) within a system; measures of intended system performance.

Pareto chart – A way of organizing data to show what major factors make up the indicator being analyzed. Useful in showing the many parts of a whole such as all the sub-indicators of a core indicator.

PDCA – Acronym for Plan-Do-Check-Act which are the four primary steps in traditional continuous quality improvement plans.

Performance Indicator – A comparison used to answer the question "how are we doing?"

Performance Measurement – The process of measuring accomplishments, as well as measuring in process parameters.

Periodic – Sampling specific data at random periods with random amounts.

Pie chart – A graphic presentation that compares relative magnitude of frequencies or parts of a whole. Useful in presenting outcome and process information.

Problem Statement: - A written description of an issue or problem which has been detected and analysed through the use of an indicator and is ready to be evaluated by a CQI group.

Population Exclusion Criteria - Specific data element/points which may be used to exclude related data from a specified data query.

GLOSSARY OF TERMS

Population Denominator (D) - The overall subject that the indicator measures.

Population Subset Numerator (N) - The subset measurement of the denominator population.

Process - The repeatable sequence of actions used throughout interrelated components of a Prehospital EMS system to produce something of value.

Process variation - Evaluations to determine if variations within a process are statistically out of control.

Published References - using published results of similar data measurements or tests as beginning or starting point for achieving or surpassing a desired goal for improvement.

Range - Maximum single data value minus the minimum single data value.

Rapid Cycle Improvement (RCI) – A form of traditional (PDCA) continuous quality improvement which emphasizes a more rapid response and change cycle.

Rate - Sampling specific data at a specific time for a specific amount.

References - Information related to the indicator which may contain helpful comparisons on indicator performance, best practices or benchmarks.

Scatter diagram - A visual display showing the relationship between two variables. Useful in showing the relationship of a process to an outcome (e.g., time & survival).

Sentinel - Sampling all specific data at all times.

Single variable - indicator end result is in a reporting value that requires only one source of data.

Six Sigma – A continuous quality improvement program which focuses primarily on evaluating data and the levels of dispersion from the bell curve means.

Source - Origin of indicator development.

Special cause - The result of a statistical trending measurement which shows a cause in variation is statistically significant and warrants further evaluation.

Standard deviation - A measurement that shows how widely spread (dispersed) any set of data is from the average.

Stratification Options - Common data elements used to stratify a specific indicator.

Structure - The interrelated components forming a Prehospital system.

Success Rate - How often a specific activity (process) is performed successfully.

Sub Indicator - Smaller indicators that are contributing factors to a core indicator.

Sub Indicator index # - Index number as classified by state EMS vision project.

Sub Indicator name - Name given to subject sub-indicator.

Trending Analysis - A series of statistical tests to determine significant variation in a process

Type of Measure - Identifies weather an indicator is structural, process, or outcome.

Variation - Evaluations to determine if a process is statistically out of control.

SUGGESTED READINGS
&
REFERENCES

SUGGESTED READINGS AND REFERENCES

1. Berwick DM: Continuous Improvement, N Engl J Medicine 320:53-56, 1989

2. Balestracci D; Data *Sanity: A Quantum Leap to Unprecedented Results, 3rd Edition.* Englewood, CO. Medical Group Management Association (MGMA), January 2009.

3. Cummings RO. The Utstein Style for uniform reporting of data for out of hospital cardiac arrest. Annals of Emerg Med. Jan 1993. 22: 37-40

4. Deming. WE: Out of Crisis. Cambridge, MASS: MIT Press International: 1982

5. Donabedian A. Definition of quality and approaches to its assessment. Ann Arbor, MI Health Administration Press; 1980

6. Donabedian A. The quality of Healthcare. JAMA. 1988: 260. 1743-1748

7. Drummond MF, Obrien BJ, Stoddard GL, Torrance GW. Methods for the economic evaluation of health programs. NY. Oxford University Press: 2003

8. Eastman JN. Walz BJ, Fear in the Workplace. Journal of EMS(JEMS) 1993: 18 (5) 53-67

9. Evans A. Avoiding Ten Benchmarking Mistakes. www.benchmarkingphs.com.ac

10. **EMSA; Emergency Medical Services System Core Quality Measures, EMSA, State of California; #166 – Appendix E, April 2013.**

11. **EMSA; Emergency Medical Services System Quality Improve Prog Model Guidelines, EMSA, State of California; #164, March 2004.**

12. **Gausche M, Lewis RJ, Stratton SJ et al. Effect on out of hospital pediatric intubation on survival and neurological outcome:. JAMA 2000; 283: 112-16**

13. **Gunderson, M; Performance Indicators, In Lerner EB, Pirrallo R, Swor R; Evaluating and Improving Quality in EMS. NAEMSP. 2009: 99-113**

14. Haynes, J: Quality Improvement in EMS: EMS WOLD EXPO; Oct 2012.

15. Institute for Healthcare Improvement' Patient Safety Development Program (IHI); Conference Handbook; Orlando, FL 2011; www. IHI.org

16. Joint Commission on Accreditation of Healthcare Organizations (JCAHO) Development and Applications of Indicators in Emergency care. 2001. 52

17. Joiner B L. *Fourth Generation Management: The New Business Consciousness.* New York, NY: McGraw-Hill, 1994 [ISBN 0-07-032715-7].

18. Mazen J. El Sayed* Measuring Quality in Emergency Medical Services: A Review of Clinical Performance Indicators; Emerg Med Int. 2012: 61630. Published online 2011 October 15. : 10.1155/2012/161630 PMCID: PMC3196253

19. Mainz J. Developing evidenced based clinical quality indicators. International Journal of Quality in Healthcare. 2003: Suppl 1: i5-i11

20. Mears G, Zalkin J, In: Kuehl A. EMS information systems and the future of EMS data base. Prehospital Emergency Care. 2001; 6: 123-130

21. Moore L. Performance Measurement in EMS. In Lerner EB, Pirrallo R, Swor R; Evaluating and Improving Quality in EMS. NAEMSP. 2009: 80-98

SUGGESTED READINGS AND REFERENCES

22. North Carolina Prehospital Medical Information Systems. www.premis.net
23. National Highway Safety Administration (NHTSA). EMS Agenda for the Future: 1996. www.nhtsa.dot.gov/people/injury/ems/agenda. Dec 4 2007.
24. National EMS Information System. www.nemsis.org
25 NHTSA Version 3.0 Uniform Data Set. 2014. www.nemsis,org
26. Sobo E, Andriese S, Stroup C, Morgan D, Kurtin P, Developing Indicators for emergency medical services (EMS) system evaluation and quality improvement; a statewide demonstration and planning project. Joint Commission; (JCAHO); Journal of Quality Improvement, 2001: 27: 138-154
27. NHTSA. Leadership Guide to Quality Improvement in EMS
28. Stickle. R: Developing a Quality Improvement Program in EMS. Advanced Leadership Issues in in EMS. Pages 9-10; http://www.usfa.fema.gov/pdf/efop/efo33925.pdf; National Fire Academy

This page left blank intentionally

Developing and Using Quality Indicators For Emergency Medical Services Evaluation and Improvement

RESOURCE APPENDIX

BI-VARIABLE INDICATOR SPECIFICATION SHEET

Measure Set	
Set Measure ID #	
Performance Measure Name	
Description	
Type of Measure	
Reporting Value	
Denominator Statement (population)	
Numerator Statement (sub-population)	
Indicator Formula Numeric Expression	
Example of Final Reporting Value	
Suggested Display Format & Frequency	
Suggested Statistical Measures	☐ Mean ☐ Median ☐ Variance ☐ Mode ☐ Standard Deviation
Trending Analysis	☐ Yes ☐ No
Benchmark Analysis	☐ Yes ☐ No
References	

DATA COLLECTION

Data Collection Approach	
Rationale for Data	
Sampling	☐ Yes ☐ No
Aggregation	☐ Yes ☐ No
Blinded	☐ Yes ☐ No
Minimum Data Values	30

DATA COLLECTION MATRIX

EMSA Core Measure ID: CAR-3										
DENOMINATOR Inclusion Criteria										
NEMSIS Element										
Field Value										
NUMERATOR Inclusion Criteria										
NEMSIS Element										
Field Value										
EXCLUSION Criteria										
NEMSIS Element										
Field Value										

SINGLE VARIABLE - INDICATOR SPECIFICATION SHEET - EXAMPLE

Measure Set	Resources
Set Measure ID #	PAD
Performance Measure Name	Public Access Defibrillation
Description	What is the number of Public Access Defibrillators in the state of California
Type of Measure	Structure
Reporting Value	Numeric
Denominator Statement (population)	Count of Defibrillator Devices
Numerator Statement (sub-population)	None
Indicator Formula Numeric Expression	Count and add the number of PAD units in California to determine total.
Example of Final Reporting Value	2087
Suggested Display Format & Frequency	Bara Graph; Data Table
Suggested Statistical Measures	☐ Mean ☐ Median ☐ Variance ☐ Mode ☐ Standard Deviation
Trending Analysis	■ Yes ☐ No
Benchmark Analysis	■ Yes ☐ No
References	AHA Standards and Guidelines for PAD programs

DATA COLLECTION

Data Collection Approach	Single variable. Make sure to count actual operating units and not programs or PAD units that are reserved or in repair.
Rationale for Data	PAD programs have been found to reduce death from out of hospital sudden cardiac arrest.
Sampling	☐ Yes ■ No
Aggregation	■ Yes ☐ No
Blinded	☐ Yes ■ No
Minimum Data Values	30

DATA COLLECTION MATRIX

EMSA Core Measure ID: CAR-3										
DENOMINATOR Inclusion Criteria	AED Units									
NEMSIS Element	D09_02									
Field Value	NA									
NUMERATOR Inclusion Criteria	None									
NEMSIS Element										
Field Value										
EXCLUSION Criteria	None									
NEMSIS Element										
Field Value										

CONTINUOUS VARIABLE - INDICATOR SPECIFICATION SHEET -EXAMPLE

Measure Set	Response Times
Set Measure ID #	RTS
Performance Measure Name	Response Time Interval
Description	What is the response time interval in mins, where 90% of all responses are equal or less than the reported value.?
Type of Measure	Process
Reporting Value	90th %
Denominator Statement (population)	All Response time intervals over a specified period of time.
Numerator Statement (sub-population)	None
Indicator Formula Numeric Expression	Rank data. Determine value at the 90th % of the ranked value. Report that value If you have 100 response times. Take and rank all of them. What is the value (mins/secs) at the 90th rank? That's you reported value.
Example of Final Reporting Value	7.8 mins
Suggested Display Format & Frequency	Run Chart; Bara Graph
Suggested Statistical Measures	☐ Mean ■ Median ☐ Variance ☐ Mode ☐ Standard Deviation
Trending Analysis	■ Yes ☐ No
Benchmark Analysis	■ Yes ☐ No
References	EMD CQI Guidelines

DATA COLLECTION

Data Collection Approach	Data must be ranked in ascending order first. What is the value which is at the 90th percentile? Formulas may be needed such as excel %.
Rationale for Data	Often reported in this format for time response compliance.
Sampling	☐ Yes ■ No
Aggregation	■ Yes ☐ No
Blinded	☐ Yes ■ No
Minimum Data Values	30

DATA COLLECTION MATRIX

EMSA Core Measure ID: CAR-3									
DENOMINATOR Inclusion Criteria	Time enrout	Time On Sce	Type Respon	Ambu resp					
NEMSIS Element	E05_05	E05_06	E03_01	E02-05					
Field Value	1990-2030	1990-2030	400-600	75					
NUMERATOR Inclusion Criteria	None								
NEMSIS Element									
Field Value									
EXCLUSION Criteria	None								
NEMSIS Element									
Field Value									

CQI INDICATOR EVALUATION FORM

INDICATOR # _____

INDICATOR TITLE: _____

	YES	NO
Does the indicator show special cause or potentially unsafe results	___	___
Is there an opportunity to increase patient safety?	___	___
Is the indicator below performance expectations?	___	___
Is there an opportunity to increase performance levels?	___	___
Is there an opportunity to institute a cost saving initiative?	___	___
Is there an opportunity to institute a operational efficiency initiative?	___	___
Does the indicator need further review or stratification?	___	___
Should an Action Plan Initiated?	___	___

Please explain any "YES" answer below;

_____

_____

_____

_____

_____

_____

LEAD REVIEWER NAME _____   DATE: _____

COMMITTEE GROUP NAME: _____

ATTACH ACTION PLAN AS INDICATED

Electronic Version Available at: _____

CQI Task Team

Problem/Issue Recognition Form

CQI Project #　　　　　_____

CQI Project Name:　　　_____

Problem/Issue Statement:

_____

_____

_____

_____

Attach appropriate documentation or supporting data as needed.

Management Leader name:　　_____

Proposed Team Leader name:　_____

Proposed Team Facilitator name: _____

Date: _____

CQI Task Team

Problem/Issue Recognition Form

Completed-Example Only

CQI Project #   <u>Initiative Project ##0125_____</u>

CQI Project Name: <u>___% Out of Hospital Cardiac Arrest</u>
<u>Survival to Hospital Discharge-2012</u>

Problem/Issue Statement:

Our CQI task Group needs to determine if our percentage (%) of cardiac arrest survival meets or exceeds the national benchmark for year 2012. The group would like to see the % survival by month for the twelve months of 2012.

References and benchmarks

Utstein Model to help determine standards and definitions..
National benchmark of 27% based upon Cardiac Arrest Registry to Enhance Survival (CARES) Q4 2012 Report

Management Leader Name: <u>Queen Elizabeth of England</u>

Proposed Team Lead name: <u>Lady Thatcher_____</u>

Proposed Team Facilitator name: <u>Secretary Clinton_____</u>

Date: <u>June 3, 2013_____</u>

CQI Task Team

Action/Implementation Plan

CQI Project #　　　　　_____

CQI Project Name:　　　_____

Improvement statement and deadlines:

_____

_____

Action Steps:　　　　　　　　　　　　Who? & by When?

❏

❏

❏

❏

❏

❏

❏

Team Leader Name:　　　_____

Team Facilitator Name:　　_____

Date:　　　　　　　_____

CQI Task Team

Action/Implementation Plan

CQI Project #   _#11453_____

CQI Project Name: Ped Med Accuracy Project_____

Improvement statement and deadlines *"Reduce the number of annual field pediatric medication errors to none (0) for a minimum of eighteen (18) consecutive months."*

Action Steps:

- ❏ To implement new tool (color coded "Broselow type" tape and county approved matching pedi medication "quick reference cards) to determine and confirm the 5 rights of the pediatric patients.

- ❏ To make pedi-med reverence tool available on both adult paramedic jump bags and in the shelves of the response units.

- ❏ Provide and communicate a clear mechanism for personnel to replace their field handbook when lost or damaged.

- ❏ Verbalize to confirm the dose and "how you got there" as a step in the administration of medications to all pedi-patients.

- ❏ Follow implementation of above changes with in-house training component.

- ❏ Explore how to integrate smart phone protocol application into work environment.

Team Leader Name: _Dr. Brilliant_____
Team Facilitator Name: _T. Anyone_____
Date: _12/14/08_____

EMS Event Report Form

Instructions: Reporting is encouraged by all who encounter an actual or potential Patient event, system concern, or exemplary care delivered that may have had an impact on the quality of care or the prevention of a potential safety event occurring within the EMS system.

      1. Inform medical personnel caring for patient as needed.
      2. Provide a concise description of the event.
      3. Submit completed form to the QI coordinator.

Please e-mail or fax this form and any attachments: EMS Fax number-01
EMS E-Mail – ems.event@EMS agency.us

EMS Use Only
Incident Type

☐ Tier 1

☐ Tier 2

☐ Tier 3

☐ Tier 4

☐ Exemplary care

☐ Other

Patient Name:	Date:
Incident/PCR#:	Time:
Initiated by (Name/Title/Organization):	
Contact Info:	Receiving Facility:
Event Location:	
Others involved with the incident. Please include name and contact info:	

Details of Event: (provide facts, observations, and statements. (Use addendum if needed) ☐ Addendum Attached

Immediate efforts to resolve this issue:

_____

_____

_____

☐ N/A
Could this event cause a community concern or a threat to public health and safety? ☐ No   ☐ Yes
If yes, contact your supervisor and the EMS Agency as soon as possible: 000-000-0000

EMS Event Form Instructions

This form is to be completed for every reported EMS event.

This information should originate from the provider involved and may be submitted anonymously

Assure that the notification process described in Policy #__ has been followed.

Provide a concise description of the event.

Individuals receiving the report should complete a brief summary of findings and disposition of the event and submit to the appropriate QI personnel.

Events that need follow-up should be conducted in coordination with QI personnel.

Oversight for the EMS event reporting process is the responsibility of each involved agency's QI staff in conjunction with the _____ County Quality Improvement Committee and EMS Agency QI Coordinator.

In reviewing the event consider the following questions

What are the facts of the events? Be objective.

What factors lead up to or contributed to the event?

What consequences resulted from the event?

Could the event been prevented? How?

What can be learned from the event?

What required actions need to be taken?

EMS Event Criteria requiring Local EMS Agency notification:

Any EMS event that leads to or has the potential to cause a community concern.

Threat to public health and safety (as defined by the Health and Safety Code 1798.200)

Any of the following actions

Fraud in the procurement of any certificate or license under this division

Gross negligence

Repeated negligent acts

Incompetence

The commission of any fraudulent, dishonest or corrupt act related to the qualification, functions and duties of prehospital personnel

Conviction of any crime which is substantially related to qualification, functions and duties of prehospital personnel

Violating or attempting to violate directly or indirectly, or assisting in or abetting the violation of or conspiring to violate, any provision of this division or regulations adopted by the authority pertaining to prehospital personnel.

Violating or attempting to violate federal or state statute or regulation which regulates narcotics, dangerous drugs or controlled substances

Addiction to the excessive use of or misuse of alcohol beverages, narcotics dangerous drugs or controlled substances

Functioning outside the supervision of medical control in the field care system operating at the local level, except as authorized by any other license or certification

Demonstration of irrational behavior or occurrence of a physical disability to the extent that a reasonable and prudent person would have reasonable cause to believe that the ability to perform the duties normally expected may be impaired.

Unprofessional conduct exhibited by any of the following

Mistreatment or physical abuse of any patient resulting from force in excess of what a reasonable and prudent person trained and acting in a similar capacity while engaged in the performance of their duties would use.

Failure to maintain confidentiality of patient medical information except as permitted by law Section 56-56.6 of the Civil Code

Commission of any sexually related offense under section 290 of the penal code.

This page left blank intentionally

Emergency Medical Services Quality Improvement Plan

Plan Template

Emergency Medical Services Quality Improvement Plan Template

Submitted by

Insert Your Provider or Agency Name

Date of Submission

This is a DRAFT COPY of a template and is intended to assist in development of a CQI plan. It does not represent nor is it sponsored, required or endorsed by any governmental, public or private entity or organization.

References:

A reference which may be helpful in developing and organizing this plan is;

California State EMS System Quality Improvement Program Model Guidelines, Publication Document#166; Section II Data Collection and Reporting for guidance on how to select these indicators. Refer to Appendix E: Indicator Categories, for indicators relative to your role in the EMS system. Refer to Appendix M: Quality Improvement Sample Indicators, for assistance identifying the indicators that relate to your organization.

www.emsa.ca.gov/pubs/pdf/emsa166.pdf

Emergency Medical Services Quality Improvement Plan

Table of Contents

Emergency Medical Services Quality Improvement Plan

I. Structure and Organizational Description

A. Describe your organizational structure, indicating your QI Program Coordinator, your Medical Director or designee (if you have one), and your internal QI structure (which may include your Medical Director or designee, QI Program Coordinator, and/or your Data Specialist). Internal QI structure may include one person or it may use an existing group in your agency/department, depending upon your agency/department's resources.

B. Describe your agency/department's external participation in the EMS System's QI Processes (for example, participation on the LEMSA QI Technical Advisory Group). Existing groups may be used to fulfill the function of your agency/department's Technical Advisory group.

C.   Describe your organization's:

•   Mission or purpose

•   Primary health care services/processes and associated standards and requirements

•   Important goals or objectives that might be specified in your strategic plan or another plan

This information should guide the remaining sections of this QI Plan and help the QI Plan reviewers understand your Plan. Please include an organization chart showing how the QI Program is integrated into the agency.

Emergency Medical Services Quality Improvement Plan

II. Data Collection and Reporting

A. Identify the specific quality indicators that your organization measures or plans to measure, including core indicators required by the .... EMS Agency. Organize your quality indicators under the following nine categories.

(1) Personnel

(2) Equipment and Supplies

(3) Documentation

(4) Clinical Care and Patient Outcome

(5) Skills Maintenance/Competency

(6) Transportation/Facilities

(7) Public Education and Prevention

(8) Risk Management

(9) Other (if not applicable to any of the other eight categories)

B. Describe the process used by your organization to select the above-listed indicators.

C. Describe how, when, and who (job title) in your organization collects data on these indicators.

D. Describe who (job title) in your organization receives reports on these indicators, on what schedule.

Emergency Medical Services
Quality Improvement Plan

III. Evaluation of Indicators

A. Describe how, how often, and who (job title) in your organization analyzes the quality indicators to enable rapid interpretation by the evaluators (Technical Advisory Group).

B. Describe or give an example of the format for presentation of quality indicator analyses (described above) to the Technical Advisory Group.
C. Describe how and when your Technical Advisory Group evaluates and makes decisions using the indicators and analyses described above.

Emergency Medical Services Quality Improvement Plan

IV. Action to Improve

A.   Describe your organization's current or planned standard approach to performance improvement. Include the steps   and sequence for action planning to improve upon results in indicators described in the previous   section.

B.   Describe how and when the Technical Advisory Group, QI Team, and   any Task Forces are involved in improvement action   planning and implementation.

C.   Describe what activities, programs, and/or systems your agency/department has in place to communicate issues regarding QI activities to involved EMS stakeholders.

D.   Describe the strategic plan or planning process used to implement changes in your organization.

Emergency Medical Services
Quality Improvement Plan

V. Training and Education

A. Describe how, how often, and who (job title) in your organization selects and provides training and to EMS staff who deliver care   to patients

B. Describe how, how often, and who (job title) in your organization standardizes needed changes emanating from improvements in policies and procedures

C. Describe how, how often, and who (job title) assures that staff successfully completes training and education required in your   QI Plan.

D. Describe the process used by your agency/department to incorporate training issues identified in the QI process into your training program.

Emergency Medical Services
Quality Improvement Plan

VI. Annual Update

The Annual Update is a written account of the progress of an organization's activities as stated in the EMS QI Program. In compiling the Annual Update, refer to the previous year's update and work plan. Describe how, how often, and who (job title) in your organization evaluates the QI Plan (annually at minimum). Annual review/updates shall include the indicators monitored, key findings/priority issues identified, improvement action plan/plans for further action, and state whether goals were met. If goals were not met, what follow-up is needed, if any?

Description of Agency

The description should include an organizational chart showing how the EMS QI Program is integrated into the organization.

Statement of EMS QI Program goals and objectives

Describe processes used in conducting quality improvement activities. Were goals and objectives met?

List and define indicators utilized during the reporting year

- Define state and local indicators
- Define provider specific indicators
- Define methods to retrieve outcome data from hospitals
- Audit critical skills
- Identify issues for further system consideration
- Identify trending issues
- Create improvement action plans
- Describe issues that were resolved
- List opportunities for improvement and plans for next cycle
- Describe continuing education and skill training provided as a result of Performance Improvement Plans
- Describe any revision of in-house policies
- Report to constituent groups
- Describe next year's work plan

About the Author

Craig Stroup is the director of the Center for Emergency Medical Services Performance Improvement and the author of many EMS articles and textbooks. He has extensive background and training in EMS systems, administration, quality improvement – especially the development and utilization of quality indicators as a powerful consensus and action tool.

With over 30 years of experience in EMS at all levels. He has been appointed and participated in many state and national EMS committees charged with developing programs and indicators for quality Improvement.
For more information or resources, Craig can be contacted at;
stroupems@msn.com

CEMSPI

Center for EMS Performance Improvement
www.cemspi.org

The Center for Emergency Medical Services (EMS) Performance improvement is a non-profit organization with the primary focus of advocating patient safety and system performance improvement specifically in the pre hospital setting.

CEMSPI works with many emergency medical services organizations to facilitate the collection, development, analysis, and maintenance of patient safety data and events reporting.

CEMSPI is also a leader in providing comprehensive quality improvement and patient safety consulting and many training options for EMS agencies and prehospital patient care providers.

Thank you to Juleine Latteri for her help with review and edit.

www.ingramcontent.com/pod-product-compliance
Lightning Source LLC
Chambersburg PA
CBHW081549170526
45166CB00009B/2628